WOMEN'S HEALTH

Robert M. Youngson

HarperCollinsPublishers

Note: Words appearing in SMALL CAPITALS are cross-references to other entries in the book which explain the term or provide additional information for the reader.

HarperCollins Publishers
P.O. Box, Glasgow G4 0NB

First published 1994

Reprint 10 9 8 7 6 5 4 3 2 1

© Robert M. Youngson 1994

ISBN 0583-33431-8

A catalogue record for this book is available
from the British Library

Printed in Great Britain

A

Amniocentesis

This is a way of finding out whether a fetus has a genetic or other disorder. The test is usually done between the 16th and 20th weeks of pregnancy. Under local anaesthesia and ultrasonic viewing, a needle is passed carefully through the wall of the abdomen and the wall of the UTERUS into the amniotic fluid in which the fetus is floating. A sample of fluid is then withdrawn. Because this fluid contains cells shed from the skin of the fetus and various substances secreted by the fetus, samples obtained contain DNA and can be of the greatest importance for diagnosis.

Alphafetoprotein levels in the amniotic fluid can give reliable information on the likelihood of congenital defects in the spinal cord and column (*spina bifida*) and absence of part of the fetal brain (*anencephaly*). Levels in the mother's blood are also measured routinely. Cells from the amniotic fluid can be grown in tissue cultures so that the chromosomes can be checked after three or four weeks. In this way, Down's syndrome and a great range of other genetic diseases, can be detected before birth. It is possible to diagnose cystic fibrosis, factor VIII and factor IX types of haemophilia, some forms of muscular dystrophy, thalassaemia, sickle cell anaemia, antitrypsin deficiency and phenylketonuria. Later in pregnancy amniocentesis provides information directly about the likelihood of a number of conditions, such as rhesus factor disease and the respiratory distress syndrome.

Amniocentesis does carry a small risk to the fetus and is not done without good reason. It may cause abortion if done early. It may damage the afterbirth (*placenta*) or the fetus and may cause bleeding into the amniotic fluid. The risk of fetal death from amniocentesis is less than 1%. Sexing of the future child is not a justification for the procedure, however anxious the future parents may be to know.

Such early methods of detection of serious or potentially serious major disorders give parents the option of an early termination of the pregnancy. They also sometimes provide the opportunity for early treatment of the disorder while the fetus remains in the uterus.

Anaemia

A reduction in the amount of the oxygen-carrying iron and protein material, haemoglobin, in the red blood cells. Because a good supply of oxygen is so vital, anaemia has widespread effects, causing weakness, fatigue, tiredness and breathlessness on minor effort. The skin may appear pale and there is lowered resistance to infection.

There are several different kinds of anaemia including simple iron deficiency anaemia, haemolytic anaemia, pernicious anaemia and aplastic anaemia. In women, by far the commonest cause is excessive menstrual loss of blood coupled with an inadequate iron intake. Anaemia may also occur because of the extra nutritional demands of pregnancy. Treatment is based on the cause and usually involves no more than supplementary iron.

Anorexia nervosa

'Anorexia' simply means 'loss of appetite' something experienced by most people from time to time. But anorexia nervosa is a serious disorder of perception that causes the sufferer, almost always a young woman, to believe that she is too fat, when, in fact, she is actually very thin. The result, inevitably, is severe emaciation. Anorexia nervosa is common in models, actresses, dancers and others who are much concerned with the appearance of their bodies. In a minority of cases it is a symptom of a serious underlying psychiatric disorder such as severe depression or schizophrenia.

The cause of anorexia is still a matter of debate. Many anorexics come from close-knit families and have a particularly intimate relationship with one parent. They are often obsessional in their habits. They are conformists and usually anxious to please. Some seem unwilling to grow up and appear to be trying to retain their childhood shape. Others seem to have a genuine fatness phobia with fear of eating fats or carbohydrates. Social factors probably contribute, especially the common and entirely arbitrary identification of slimness with sexual attractiveness. Such influences may powerfully affect girls who are deeply concerned with how they are regarded by others.

Medically, the effects of anorexia nervosa, often hidden by the sufferer in the early stages, are obvious. The signs of starvation are unfortunately only too clear. When calorie intake is less than energy expenditure and the needs of structural replacement, first the fat stores are used up and then the muscles are used for fuel. In anorexia there is extreme thinness with loss of a third or more of the body weight. There is, inevitably, severe tiredness and weakness and often the effects of vitamin deficiency. The skin becomes dry and the hair falls out. Early in the process there is, in almost all cases, absence of menstruation. Death from starvation, or suicide, is common.

Anorexia nervosa demands skilled treatment in hospital under the care of those experienced in the condition. Personality problems and the persistence of the disorder can make treatment difficult. Management depends on psychotherapy and insistence on re-feeding. Patients will usually make every effort to circumvent treatment, holding food in their mouths until it can be disposed of. Strict control is essential. Unless a watch is kept, food will be hidden or secretly thrown away. Often a system of rewards may be effective, in which privileges, such as visits or leave passes, are awarded for weight gained.

Antidepressant drugs are often helpful in the early stages. Even after normal weight has been regained, young women who have had anorexia nervosa may need to remain under psychiatric care for months or years. Relapses are common and, tragically, up to 10% later die from suicide or starvation.

Anxiety

Anxiety is a natural response to threat or danger, whether real or imagined. When people are anxious their bodies produce certain hormones, which, while helping to cope with the danger, also cause some very unpleasant symptoms.

The persistently worried state of mind involves being constantly 'keyed up'. This causes:

- an exaggerated startle response
- lack of concentration
- irritability
- insomnia
- a tendency for the mind to 'go blank'

Closely related to these mental effects are the corresponding physical manifestations. These are many, and include:

- a rapid pulse
- muscle tension
- tooth-grinding (*bruxism*)
- restlessness
- easy fatiguability
- breathlessness
- tremulousness
- palpitations
- a feeling of tightness in the chest
- sweating
- clammy hands
- dry mouth
- nausea
- diarrhoea
- flushing
- frequency of urination
- a 'lump in the throat'

There is narrowing of attention and reduced mental efficiency with disorganisation and poor performance. Doctors are still arguing whether these symptoms are the effect of the state of mind or are the cause of it.

ANXIETY

Severe anxiety that occurs without any obvious cause is abnormal, disabling and very common. Terms describing such states quickly become derogatory and some doctors, for reasons of sympathy, keep changing them. Anxiety states or anxiety neuroses have become *free-floating* anxiety. Hypochondriasis has become a *psychosomatic disorder*. And phobias have become *situational anxiety*.

Anxiety often seems deeply rooted in the personality. Many anxious people are convinced that their symptoms are due to organic disease. The physical symptoms of anxiety help to promote the belief that there is heart disease, cancer or AIDS. These unfortunate people often undergo repeated and fruitless medical investigation. Some become psychologically dependent on doctors who are kind to them and on tranquillizing drugs. They do not always get effective treatment.

Many of the symptoms of anxiety can be relieved. Beta blockers and antihistamine drugs are often very effective. The benzodiazepine drugs like Valium and Librium were once widely used, but their disadvantages – dependency and addiction – are now apparent and they are being replaced by newer 'anxiolytic' drugs, for which better things are claimed. Tricyclic and monoamine oxidase inhibiting antidepressant drugs have some part to play in the treatment of anxiety.

Anxiety may also be a symptom of various other conditions including thyroid overactivity (see THYROID GLAND DISORDERS), menopausal hormonal disturbances, drug withdrawal, schizophrenia, depressive illness, post-concussional syndrome and dementia. Long-term anxiety, however, is unlikely to be due to organic disorder.

B

Backache

Lumbago, or low back pain, is one of the commonest and most persistent of symptoms. It is especially common in pregnancy and following childbirth. The idea that backache is caused by a turned-back (*retroverted*) uterus is no longer believed. Most cases are due to faulty posture and to the maintenance, after pregnancy, of the forward bend in the lower spine (*lordosis*), which is an inevitable feature of late pregnancy. Cases caused in this way will usually clear up soon after delivery, especially if attention is given to the posture.

It is a mistake, however to assume that backache is necessarily associated with pregnancy. Many cases occur at other times. The symptom becomes more frequent with age, and about half of all those over sixty suffer frequently from it. In most of these cases it is also due to a defective, slouching posture associated with poor development in the large group of muscles surrounding the spine (*paravertebral muscles*). Backache caused in this way can usually be relieved by exercises to strengthen the muscles and by the adoption of a proper, upright posture, both in standing and in sitting. Often, this type of backache is brought on, or made worse, by obesity or by unaccustomed or injudicious work or weight-bearing.

The fibrous connective tissue of the back muscles, ligaments and tendons is often the site of pain and this may follow unusual or strenuous exercise, especially in sport in the untrained. Lumbar pain can also be related to mental stress, virus infections, sleep disorders and anxiety.

BACKACHE

The most common serious form of back pain is caused by what is popularly described as 'slipped disc'. This is an inaccurate term as the discs between the bodies of the vertebrae of the spine are very securely attached to the bone and cannot slip. Even the official medical term – prolapsed intervertebral disc – is not quite right. It is not the disc that is displaced, but a variable quantity of the soft, pulpy central material (*nucleus pulposus*) which is forced by longitudinal pressure through a localized defect in the outer fibrous ring of the disc and squashed backwards to press on the spinal nerves. Pressure on these nerves causes, not only severe backache, but also pain which radiates down the course of the nerve – through the buttock, back of the thigh and down as far as the foot. These nerves are bundled together to form the main nerve trunk supplying the leg (*sciatic nerve*) and pressure on them causes not only severe backache but sciatica. Severe backache and stiffness associated with involvement of the sciatic nerve – pain, numbness or loss of function – indicate a prolapsed disc and call for proper medical or surgical treatment.

There are many other causes of backache, but these are much less common. They include:

- a tear of a muscle or ligament
- an actual fracture of one of the facets or processes of a vertebra
- wearing away of the joint surfaces (*chronic osteoarthritis*)
- inflammation of the spine (*ankylosing spondylitis*)
- minor abnormalities of the lower part of the spine present from birth (congenital bone defects)
- a slipping forward of the lowest lumbar vertebra on the top of the sacrum (*spondylolisthesis*)

- bone tuberculosis
- bone marrow cancer (*myeloma*) or secondary cancer which has spread to the bone

Most attacks of acute low back pain settle in a few days, but it is important to try to determine and avoid the cause as, otherwise, recurrence is likely. This may lead to a permanent (*chronic*) situation. In severe and persistent cases it is essential to seek medical advice so that a correct diagnosis can be reached and appropriate treatment given. Backache is a *symptom* – an indication of something else, not a disease in its own right.

Osteopaths believe that many backaches are caused by actual displacement of one vertebra relative to another and that they can be relieved by identifying the site of the dislocation and applying pressure to reduce it. Certainly, many people have been relieved of their backache by osteopathic treatment, but most doctors are sceptical of the claimed cause. A good osteopath will probably know more about backache than most doctors, but there is always the worry that treatment will be undertaken without an accurate diagnosis. This can be dangerous, if only by delaying access to proper management.

Blushing

Blushing is a transient reddening of the face, ears and neck, often spreading to the upper part of the chest, but rarely, if ever, to more remote parts of the body. The skin contains an extensive network of small arteries with smooth muscle fibres in their walls. Normally, these muscles are in a state of partial contraction. Extreme contraction causes the arteries to close down so that less blood flows through the skin and it becomes pale. Full relaxation of these muscles causes widening of the blood vessels and a larger quantity of blood than normal passes through the skin causing flushing, or blushing.

These tiny artery muscles are controlled by nerves of the non-voluntary (*autonomic*) nervous system and this, in turn, is affected by various influences, including the emotions. Any strong tendency to blush, as in adolescence, may thus be due both to emotional instability and to undue sensitivity of the autonomic system. Adolescent blushing commonly ceases to be a problem with maturity and growing social confidence.

Widening of blood vessels is a feature of sexual excitement, especially in women, and a widespread mottled flush commonly occurs during sexual intercourse. The hot flushes of the menopause are also caused by blood vessels widening. In this case, the stimulus to the autonomic system is a deficiency of the female sex hormone, oestrogen.

Blushing can become a permanent problem. The disease acne rosacea (not to be confused with common acne) is a state of permanent widening of the blood vessels of the skin of the cheeks and nose. There are effective treatments for this condition.

Breast abscess

Breast inflammation (*mastitis*) is common during breastfeeding because the nipples often suffer injury and abrasion. Germs pass into the breast by way of these abrasions and set up an infection. There is painful swelling in the affected breast, redness, tenderness, tension and often inability to pass milk. Soon the breast becomes extremely swollen, there is fever and general upset and the lymph nodes in the armpit swell and become tender. General breast tenderness and tension are normal features of the first few days of lactation, but any local tenderness, redness or pain must be reported at once.

Mastitis that is not properly treated with antibiotics may rapidly progress to abscess, but this may occur even if antibiotics are given. One or more areas of softening and local tissue destruction occur and collections of pus form. At this stage a minor surgical operation is necessary to open abscesses and release the pus. Milk production must be stopped with hormones.

Breast cancer

This is the commonest form of cancer in women and a very common disease, affecting about one woman in 14 in Britain. It is the leading cause of death among women between 40 and 55 years of age in the USA. In Japan, by contrast, the incidence is only about one fifth that in the USA. The medical literature on the subject is enormous and many hundreds, if not thousands of trials of all kinds, connected with the disease, have been done. As a result statistics on breast cancer are very complicated and sometimes contradictory. It is difficult to get entirely reliable figures and any quoted here should be taken as only approximate.

Breast cancer is rare before the age of 30 and the incidence rises rapidly during the 40s. After the menopause, the incidence continues to rise with age, but less rapidly. About one third of cases occur under the age of 50, one third between 50 and 64 and one third in women over 64. The risk of breast cancer is doubled if the mother had it, and is increased about three times in those who have already had it in one breast. Again, figures are uncertain and vary with the individual. Other less important risk factors are believed to be:

- having no children
- starting menstruation early
- exposure to radiation
- being in a high socioeconomic group
- eating a high-fat diet
- taking large doses of oestrogens
- taking oral contraceptives
- tallness
- alcohol intake
- having had cancer of the ovaries or of the lining of the UTERUS.

The risk is believed to be doubled in women who habitually drink three units of alcohol a day. Women with many children and those who have had their ovaries removed (*oophorectomy*) are less likely, than average, to get breast cancer.

Breast cancers are insidious and hardly ever cause pain. There may, sometimes, be a vague discomfort, but, commonly, the only sign is the finding of a slowly growing lump. There are, however, other possible signs and these should be known and looked for. They are:

- distortion of the normal breast contour by skin dimpling
- indrawing, or alteration in direction, of the nipple
- bleeding from the nipple
- distortion of the area around the nipple (*areola*)
- orange-skin texture appearance (*peau d'orange*) of the breast skin

- alteration in the position or hang of the breast compared to the other side
- rubbery, firm, easily felt glands (lymph nodes) in the armpit

Breast cancer can spread directly, or by passing along lymph channels, to and through the lymph nodes or even by way of the bloodstream. Remote spread is usually to the lungs, bones and liver. Minimal breast cancers are those confined to the milk ducts and lobes of the breast. They remain in the original location (*in situ*) for a long time before becoming invasive and spreading outside the breast and are easily curable if detected. They nearly always occur in pre-menopausal women. Unfortunately they do not produce a swelling that can be felt and are almost always detected at pathological examination for cancer suspected for other reasons – such as innocent fibrosis or cysts. Rarely, minimal cancers of this kind may become chalky (*calcified*) and may be detected by high-grade special X-ray examination (*mammography*).

The diagnosis of breast cancer is by microscopic examination by a pathologist, of tissue from the lump. This is called a biopsy and the tissue may be obtained by cutting into the breast and removing suspect tissue under direct inspection, or by sucking out some cells through a needle. The significance and probable outcome of breast cancer depend on the stage the tumour has reached when discovered. The size of the cancer is one of the most important factors. With tumours less than 2 cm across at the time of diagnosis and treatment, 60% of women are free of recurrences five years later. If tumours are 2–5 cm across, about 45% of the women are free of recurrence at five years. But for tumours more than 5 cm across, only about 20% of women are free of recurrence. This highlights the importance of monthly self-examination (see BREAST, SELF-EXAMINATION). Several careful studies have shown that tumour size is substantially and significantly less, at the time of diagnosis in women who practice regular self-examination.

Mammography as a screening method for breast cancer has greatly improved in reliability in recent years and the dosage of radiation has been reduced so that it is not now believed to be a hazard. Experts now believe that mammography, if properly done, can reduce the mortality from BREAST cancer by one-third in women over 50.

The outlook in breast cancer is worsened if the cancer has spread to the lymph nodes in the armpit, and greatly worsened if there are discernible distant outgrowths of tumour (*metastases*). Delay in seeking investigation and treatment is therefore most dangerous. Several studies have shown that women who delay for more than three months after finding a lump, subsequently proved to be cancer, have a substantially lower survival rate then those who report the problem within three months. This fact should be known to all women, and used, if necessary as a basis for protest against medical delays. You must never delay on the grounds of fright or shyness.

Women not treated at all do very badly. Conventional treatment of breast cancer has, in the past, been mainly by radical mastectomy–surgical removal of all breast tissue and the connected lymph nodes together with the removal of the underlying chest muscles (*pectorals*). As a rough approximation, the five-year survival rate has been about 50% overall. For those without lymph node involvement, the rate has been about 70% and for those with lymph node cancer, about 30%.

It has to be stated, however, that breast cancer can spread remotely even without involvement of the glands in the armpit. This and other factors led surgeons to pay less attention to radical and mutilating operations and more to the possibility of treatment by more limited surgery combined with various combinations of radiotherapy, anti-cancer chemotherapy, hormone treatment and immune system boosting. Radical surgery is now usually restricted to total removal of the breast and lymph tissues with preservation of the muscles. This gives much improved appearance and function and makes breast reconstruction easier. In recent years there has been a trend towards even less mutilating operations and it is now common to employ a simple removal of the mass (*lumpectomy*) followed by a course of radiotherapy using linear accelerators or a cobalt-60 source.

The study of the results of such methods shows that they are no worse than those of radical mastectomy and that cancerous nodes can be treated just as effectively by radiation as by operation. A great many clinical trials have been done to compare the effectiveness of various regimes of treatment for cancer that has spread beyond the breast. But the possible permutations and combinations of different methods and different groups, in terms of cancer stage, are so great that the results are difficult to interpret. Moreover, not all present methods of cancer treatment have been available long enough for the long-term outcome to be known. We do know, however, that chemotherapy substantially reduces the mortality in pre-menopausal women with cancer that has spread to the lymph nodes in the armpit. Hormonal therapy has been found most useful in cases where the cancer has spread widely. Immune system therapy is recent and promising.

Traditionally, the treatment of breast cancer has been the province of the general surgeon. This is no longer considered appropriate. Breast cancer is a speciality in its own right calling for specialized knowledge and skills. The results of treatment by such specialists are significantly better than those of most general surgeons. This fact has recently been recognized by the British government and new guidelines for the setting up of specialized cancer centres have been published.

See also BREAST LUMP, BREAST RECONSTRUCTION, BREAST REMOVAL, TAMOXIFEN.

Breast leakage

This is called galactorrhoea, which means, literally, 'a flowing of milk'. The term is used to indicate an excessive flow, or spontaneous production of milk at times when lactation should not be occurring. Milk supply can be kept up almost indefinitely if the stimulus of suckling continues, but once this is removed, lactation ceases.

Galactorrhoea can occur in both women and men and even in babies. About 30% of the cells of the front half of the pituitary gland are prolactin hormone-producing cells; a tumour of these, a prolactinoma, will secrete large quantities of the hormone and promote a flow of milk from the breasts. Unexplained galactorrhoea in an adult is thus an important sign of a possibly serious condition – a pituitary gland tumour – and should never be ignored. Galactorrhoea may also occur as a side-effect of certain drugs. Just before birth, babies are exposed to concentrations of this hormone in the maternal blood and often show some milk production – *witches milk* – for a few days after birth. This is quite normal and harmless.

Breast inflammation

The medical term for this is mastitis. This is commonest during the period of milk production (*lactation*) and is usually caused by infection with germs that get in through cracks or abrasions in the nipples. Mastitis is especially likely if the baby has a skin infection. It causes high fever, local redness, pain, tenderness and hardening, and, unless the infection is successfully controlled by early antibiotic treatment, an abscess may form which may have to be opened and drained surgically.

The term *chronic mastitis* is sometimes applied to a condition in which the breasts are of an irregular rubbery consistency and contain painful or tender nodules or cysts. This is not an inflammation and the condition, which is common, is not a mastitis. It is related to the balance of the hormones which control the menstrual cycle and does not normally require treatment.

Breast lump

All breasts are naturally lumpy as they contain glandular tissue and this normal lumpiness is often more obvious just before a menstrual period. Sometimes what seems to be a new swelling is felt before a period. Such a swelling is often tender or painful but disappears after the end of menstruation. This kind of swelling is most unlikely to be serious.

The term 'breast lump' refers to an isolated, usually painless, swelling. Such a lump, which does not become more prominent before a period and which does not disappear afterwards, should always be regarded as potentially serious and should be reported without delay. Most breast lumps – about 75% – are entirely benign and are due either to BREAST INFLAMMATION, a breast cyst, or a non-malignant breast tumour. But breast cancer *is* common and if you are in any doubt you should regard this as a reason for reporting the lump, not for delaying (see BREAST CANCER).

BREAST SELF-EXAMINATION is an obvious precaution and should be done every month. Contrary to common belief, breast cancers are often entirely painless, so you will not know you have a lump unless you feel it, or leave it to a dangerously late stage. Don't, on any account, be put off by fear. If the doctor thinks the lump is suspicious, the chances are that all that will happen is that a few cells from it will be sucked out through a fine needle. This is called a needle biopsy and is nothing to worry about. The cells will quickly be examined under the microscope. What happens after that depends on the pathologist's findings. *Never* delay reporting a breast lump. You should protest strenuously if there is any medical delay after you have reported it. Quote government policy.

Breast reconstruction

Women who have had to have a breast removed, usually because of cancer, present quite different problems from those who simply need breast reduction. Here, the requirement is for the more complicated process of breast reconstruction. Today, breast cancer surgery is often less extensive than it used to be, and reconstruction operations are correspondingly easier. But radical mastectomy, in which all breast tissue and often the underlying muscles too, are removed, leaves a woman sadly mutilated. The reconstitution of a symmetrical breast, in such a case, is difficult and may involve both tissue transplantation and plastic augmentation. But women who have had to have a breast removed deserve the sympathetic attention of the surgeon, and usually get it. Most women who have lost a breast are depressed and anxious and feel sexually disadvantaged. If you have had a breast removed and are distressed by the mutilation, you should certainly see whether something can be done to help.

It is undeniably harder to get a good result, and especially a good match in size and shape, when a breast and the underlying muscles have been removed.

In reconstruction operations the difficulty is always to achieve adequate symmetry. If the other breast is large, the reconstructed breast is likely to be too small and the question then arises as to whether a reduction operation, on the normal breast, is justified. This will, of course, mean more scars and you may feel that you already have enough of those. A perfect result is impossible and you should understand the limitations of breast reconstruction. If you feel you have real doubts about the project you may be best to abandon the idea.

It is usual to defer breast reconstruction until three months to a year after the breast removal operation. The longer period is advisable if you have had radiotherapy, which interferes with sound healing and increases the chances of graft rejection. Some surgeons, however, will undertake reconstruction at the time of the original mastectomy operation.

Simple mastectomy without removal of the pectoral muscles is usually adequately dealt with by a straightforward breast augmentation. But if you have had a radical mastecto-my, both the skin and the underlying tissue bulk must be replaced. The operation will always be performed under general anaesthesia.

The commonest and safest site from which the necessary tissue can be taken is from your back. Just under the skin of your upper back, on either side, is a thick, broad muscle. So long as the incision is made in the direction in which the muscle fibres run – sloping up towards your shoulder from the midline – a fairly large elliptical piece of skin with attached underlying muscle, together with its blood supply, can safely be brought to the front. If the blood supply is preserved, the chances of a successful graft are very high. The edges of the cut muscle and skin are brought together with stitches. The donated skin allows the necessary increase in skin area for the new breast and the muscle helps to increase the bulk. It is not feasible to remove enough muscle to produce an adequately sized breast so an additional silicone implant is used to make up the deficit.

An alternative donor site is the front of the abdomen. Here, there is usually plenty of skin and underlying fat. When this site is used an implant may be unnecessary. In some cases, using this site has the added advantage that the procedure gets rid of an unwanted abdominal bulge and helps to produce a slimmer figure. The disadvantage is that there is a greater risk that the graft will fail to take. The loss of muscle from the abdominal wall can also lead later to hernia development.

The surgeon's final problem is to produce an artificial nipple. This is also difficult and, if done, is usually deferred for about three months. The areola can be simulated by a disc of skin taken from the inside of the thigh and the remaining nipple can be split to provide nipple tissue if it is large enough. Alternatively, an ear lobe, or a disc of skin taken from elsewhere, can be used. By this stage, many women feel they have had enough surgery and prefer to use an adhesive artificial nipple.

Breast removal

Surgical removal of the breast is called mastectomy. This is done almost exclusively for the treatment of cancer.

Radical mastectomy, now much less often done than formerly, involves the removal of all breast tissue and breast skin, the underlying pectoral muscles and the lymph nodes in the armpit. This involves a large, elliptical cut sloping diagonally down from the armpit to the lower part of the centre of the chest.

In simple mastectomy, only the breast tissue is removed. An elliptical cut around the nipple is used and it is sometimes possible to restore a reasonably realistic appearance with an implant. The general trend, today, is to an even less radical procedure called *lumpectomy* in which only the obvious mass is removed through a short radial cut. Ancillary treatment to reduce the chances of regrowth or recurrence of the cancer is essential.

Breast self-examination

BREAST CANCER is the commonest form of cancer in women. Contrary to common belief, it is often entirely painless. There may sometimes be vague discomfort, but usually the only sign is a slowly growing lump. So unless you or someone else deliberately looks for it, the chances are that breast cancer will not be detected until a dangerously late stage. For any woman with breast cancer the outlook depends critically on how long the cancer has been present when it is discovered.

Clinical examination by a doctor, and especially the kind of X-ray screening known as MAMMOGRAPHY, are valuable. Mammography can detect small cancers less than 1 cm across. If there is a family history of breast cancer or any other indication, or if you are over 50, regular mammography combined with frequent examination give the best chance.

No doctor can be as familiar with the normal feel of your breasts as you are, and you can with very little inconvenience carry out the examination once a month. There is really no substitute for regular monthly self-examination and if you don't do it you may regret it. If you are still menstruating, you should examine your breasts every month during the week after your period. It is normal for your breasts to be lumpy during and just before the periods and it is more difficult then to know what you are feeling. If your periods have stopped, do the examination on a particular date – such as the first day of every month.

Here is a good routine: strip to the waist and stand straight in front of a large mirror with your arms hanging loose. Check that your breasts are of exactly the usual shape, size and colour. Check both nipples for any change in their position, relative to the rest of the breast and to one another and look carefully for any indrawing or any sign of dimpling. Check for bleeding from the nipples. Gently squeeze around each nipple to see whether you can express any discharge from the nipple itself. Look at the breast contours and check especially for puckering of the skin or an appearance like orange skin. Always compare the two sides. They need not be identical – indeed breasts seldom are – but any alteration in the usual difference may be important. Raise your arms equally above your head and check the lower parts of your breasts. See whether they move up equally when you raise your arms. Look especially to see whether one seems to be tethered or held down.

Now lie on your back so that the muscles under your breasts are relaxed and feel both breasts for lumps. Some women find it easier with a folded towel behind the shoulder-blade on the side of the breast being examined. Use your right hand for the left breast and your left hand for the right. Feel only with the flat of your fingers. Do not pinch the breast tissue between fingers and thumb – it will always feel lumpy if you do it this way. Work around each breast systematically, checking each of the four quadrants and the tail of the breast which points up to the armpit. This is called the axillary tail and is especially important as many tumours occur here. Don't forget to feel carefully for lumps in the armpit. Throughout, you are searching for a firm, hardish swelling which may or may not move freely. But you are also looking for any change, however slight. If you have any suspicion of anything new, report it to your doctor at once. Delay may be dangerous.

Broken veins

This term is inaccurate and misleading. The medical word for the condition, however – *telangiectasia* – is likely to tell you even less. This appearance is due to localized widening of small veins near the surface of the skin. It is one of the natural features of the ageing skin and the cause is simply loss of support of the vessels from a reduction in the amount of the skin protein collagen. In most people, the amount of collagen in the skin declines progressively with age. Telangiectasia, which is made worse by alcohol excess and undue exposure to sun and cold, is of cosmetic importance only.

A condition called rosacea, a sort of BLUSHING disorder, features widespread telangiectasia. This condition, although nothing to do with infection, responds well to regular small doses of the antibiotic tetracycline. Telangiectasia can also be caused by frequent use of steroid preparations on the skin.

Some people are sufficiently distressed by telangiectasia to submit to destruction of the affected parts of the vessels by freezing (*cryotherapy*), electrolysis, laser treatment or electrocoagulation. This may leave small scars and recurrence is likely. The laser is probably the most effective method.

Bulimia

Bulimia is an uncontrollable, compulsive eating disorder usually affecting intelligent young women and causing them to eat large quantities of food in a very short period of time. As many as 15,000 Calories may be taken in a few hours. In spite of this, those affected are seldom overweight and most of them appear normal. In many, the weight varies at an abnormal rate, fluctuating above and below the ideal. Friends and relatives often do not suspect bulimia because the *binge eating* and the behaviour that follows are usually kept secret. Binge episodes are often triggered by mental or social stress.

Women with bulimia can't help themselves and regularly eat to the point of bloating and nausea. These binges may, in mild cases, occur only once every few weeks, and, in such cases, strict dieting, in between episodes, is enough to keep the weight down. But in other cases, the cycle takes place every day or even several times a day. These unfortunate young women have to find a private place for their activities because the binges are followed by regret and a panicky concern that the result will be a gain in weight. So they deliberately cause themselves to vomit and take purgatives, to empty the bowel and undo the 'harm'. Some young women even take drugs, known as diuretics, which cause excessive output of urine and temporary loss of weight until the resulting thirst forces them to drink and replace the deficient fluid.

The physical problems with bulimia are caused by repeated vomiting and laxative and diuretic use, which may reduce the normal acidity of the blood and upset the balance of dissolved substances even to the extent of causing muscular weakness or the state of muscular spasm called tetany. There may be persistently sore throat and heartburn from the vomited acid, and the salivary glands in the cheeks may be inflamed in a manner similar to mumps. Teeth may be badly damaged, even reduced to sharp stumps, by the repeated action of stomach acid and the knuckles may be scarred from the attempts to force the fingers down the throat to induce vomiting.

On the psychological side, up to half the cases of bulimia have features in common with ANOREXIA NERVOSA. Women with anorexia, have a distorted image of their own bodies, and in

25

spite of the evidence of the mirror, are deeply preoccupied with becoming too fat. Most cases of bulimia, however, are caused by a less serious psychological upset than anorexia, and treatment, by specialists in the disorder, is generally more successful. Bulimia is not just a matter of self-control but is a recognized medical condition for which medical help is needed.

C

Caesarean section

This is an operation, often performed in a hurry, to remove a baby from the UTERUS of a pregnant woman through an incision in the front wall of the abdomen. In ancient Rome, the operation was commonly performed immediately after the death of a woman near term. Numa Pompilius (762–715 BC) passed a law requiring that the fetus was to be cut out when a woman died in labour. This became the *Lex Caesarea* and it is likely that this is the origin of the term.

Today, Caesarean section is an indispensable procedure and has become very safe. It is done whenever delay in delivery threatens the life of the baby or the mother, or when normal delivery would be dangerous for the child. Common indications for performing the operation are:

- heartbeat changes in the fetus (*fetal distress*)
- an afterbirth (*placenta*) placed near the exit of the UTERUS (*placenta praevia*)
- the appearance of the umbilical cord before the baby
- a baby that is too large for the woman's pelvis (*disproportion*)
- breech presentation
- an excessively large baby caused by diabetes in the mother
- danger to the baby from blood breakdown (*haemolytic disease of the newborn*) resulting from rhesus incompatibility

- uncontrollable high blood pressure in the mother (*pre-eclampsia*)
- failure of the UTERUS to contract properly
- bleeding (*antepartum haemorrhage*)

The operation is performed under general, epidural or spinal anaesthesia. The incision is made, vertically or transversely, well below the navel, the bladder is pushed down off the uterus and a short transverse cut is made into the lower part of the uterus and carefully deepened until the internal, fluid-filled membranes begin to bulge through. These are left intact initially and the incision is enlarged sideways, usually by pulling with the fingers, until it is wide enough to allow the baby to get out. The membranes are now ruptured and the head delivered, followed by the body. The placenta soon separates and is removed. The wall of the uterus is closed with absorbable catgut or other stitches and the abdominal wound is closed in layers.

Cancer screening

The commonest cancers in women are those of the breast, large bowel (*colon* and *rectum*), and, increasingly, lung. Some success has been achieved in the efforts to screen for breast cancer and the results have been most encouraging. In the USA a group of 20,000 women aged 40 to 64 were checked by careful examination of the breasts and by the special X-ray test, MAMMOGRAPHY. The mortality rate was reduced by 30% in comparison with an exactly equivalent group of women who were not screened. Ten years after the trial had started, there had been 97 deaths from breast cancer in the screened group and 137 deaths from the same cause in the unscreened group. About one third of the breast cancers detected by mammography were in the early stage before they had invaded other tissues.

BREAST SELF-EXAMINATION is an important form of screening and every woman should be familiar with the signs indicating the need for immediate medical attention.

Cancers of the large bowel frequently produce very slight bleeding, not sufficient to appear as visible blood in the stools, but sufficient to be detected by a sensitive test using paper impregnated with a chemical indicator. Trials, using this method have been reported in *The Lancet* and are accepted by about half of those to whom they are offered. It is not yet quite clear whether this is a worthwhile method. Individual awareness is essential. Blackening of the stool, from the iron in released haemoglobin, frank blood in the stools, changes in the bowel habit, unexplained and severe constipation – indeed, almost any unusual feature – should alert you to the possibility that something serious may be wrong.

Regrettably, screening for lung cancer has not been a great success. This is not because the methods are ineffective. Four-monthly chest X-rays and sputum tests can detect almost 90% of cases. But the class of people at greatest risk – young smokers of the lower socioeconomic groups – have been found to be unwilling to take advantage of such screening methods. The indications are that the money would be better spent in trying to promote measures to discourage smoking.

Cervical erosion

This is an inaccurate term that describes a raw appearance of the outer part of the neck of the UTERUS (*cervix*). In fact, the appearance is caused by a perfectly normal extension of the inner lining (*endocervix*) out on to the usually smooth and lighter-coloured covering membrane. The extension of this velvety red area on to the cervix is especially common during pregnancy when the high levels of oestrogen promote growth of the lining of the canal of the cervix. Occasionally there is a slight mucus, or sometimes bloodstained, discharge.

Not many years ago, it was common to attribute all sorts of symptoms to cervical erosion and many treatments, especially cauterization, were given. Nowadays, gynaecologists know better, and so long as a CERVICAL SMEAR TEST shows no abnormality the condition is usually ignored. Occasionally it may cause vaginal discharge or bleeding after intercourse. In these cases treatment may be needed.

Cervical smear test

A screening test used to detect early cancer of the neck of the UTERUS (*cervix*). It was developed by George Nicholas Papanicolaou (1883–1962), an American pathologist of Greek origin, working at Cornell Medical College, New York. Cancer of the cervix is preventable if detected at the stage known as *carcinoma in situ* or *intra-epithelial neoplasia*. At this stage the cancerous changes in the cells (*neoplasia*) have begun, but the process is still confined to the lining (*epithelium*) and has not spread deeper. The test is performed on over three million women a year in Britain and, as a result, there has been a striking increase in the number found to have these early changes.

The 'Pap test', as it is called in the USA, is an example of *exfoliative cytology* – a technique in which isolated cells are examined microscopically by a skilled pathologist and suspicious changes noted. The Pap smear is simple. The skill lies in the interpretation of changes in the cells. A metal or plastic instrument (*speculum*) is gently inserted to keep the vagina open and a small, blunt-edged plastic or wooden spatula is used to scrape some cells gently from in and around the opening of the cervix. These are then smeared on a microscope slide, stained and examined.

The pathologist may find signs of inflammation from *Trichomonas vaginalis*, THRUSH, herpes and other infections. But he or she is primarily concerned with the characteristic cell changes caused by the human papillomavirus – a cavity near the nucleus, or a doubling or unusually deep staining of the nuclear (*chromosomal*) material. These changes are present in over 80% of cases showing suspicion of malignancy. The earliest stage of possible malignant change is shown by cells with abnormal, usually enlarged, nuclei. This is called *dyskaryosis*.

Cytology is very difficult and can be done successfully only by experienced pathologists. Because of this difficulty, the failure to detect abnormality (false negative rate), in the very earliest stage, is admitted to be 10–15%. But cytology can detect nearly all cases of established carcinoma *in situ*. These facts emphasize the importance of repeated testing, especially if you have already had an abnormal smear result. In some centres, checks have shown, unfortunately, that only about 60% of women with abnormal smears attend for follow-up.

Ideally, three-yearly screening should be carried out on all sexually active women over 35, women who have been pregnant three or more times and women who present for contraceptive advice. Women with abnormal smears are treated by cervical freezing, high-frequency cautery (*electrodiathermy*) or laser evaporation. One treatment gives a cure rate of 95%.

Cervicitis

This is inflammation of the neck of the UTERUS (*cervix*). Most cases of cervicitis are caused by sexually transmitted organisms, especially:

- *Chlamydia trachomatis*, which causes *non-specific urethritis*
- the gonococcus, which causes gonorrhoea
- *Herpes simplex* virus, type II, which causes venereal herpes

Often, the condition causes no symptoms, but there may be a vaginal discharge and, if infection has spread more widely, sometimes pain on intercourse. The organisms concerned often also cause urinary symptoms, such as frequency and a burning pain on urination.

The condition responds well to antibiotics, but sexual partners should also be checked and treated. It is best to avoid unprotected sexual intercourse until treatment is complete.

Chlamydial infections

Infections with organisms of the *Chlamydial* genus, especially *Chlamydia trachomatis*, can cause widespread infection of the genital tract in women, and commonly lead to:

- inflammation of the neck of the UTERUS (CERVICITIS)
- inflammation and blockage of the fallopian tubes (*salpingitis*)
- inflammation of the glands that produce sexual lubricant mucus (*Bartholinitis*)

These infections are usually sexually transmitted. Chlamydia is now the commonest of the sexually transmitted diseases in Britain and USA. Inflammatory blockage of the FALLOPIAN TUBES is a common cause of infertility.

Chloasma

A mask-like area of brownish coloration, involving the skin around the eyes, nose, cheeks and forehead, which often affects women during pregnancy or when taking oral contraceptives. Chloasma sometimes occurs after the menopause. It tends to be worse if the skin is exposed to sunlight. The pigmentation usually fades in time.

Clitoris

This is the female version of the penis and, like the penis, is an erectile organ. It is the main centre of erotic sensitivity and has plenty of sensory nerves. The clitoris varies greatly in size from one woman to another. Its most sensitive part, the glans, or tip, is partly hooded by a fold of skin called the prepuce. This fold is connected to the labia minora. During vaginal intercourse, effective movements by the man cause this fold to massage the glans of the clitoris. If arousal is sufficient, this massage is likely to lead to clitoral erection and orgasm. Many women do not experience clitoral stimulation in this way and more direct stimulation may be needed. See also SEXUAL PROBLEMS.

Colposcopy

The direct microscopic examination of the surface of the neck of the UTERUS (*cervix*). The microscope has a long focus so that it can be used well outside the vulva and the vagina is held open by a kind of spreader called a speculum. Colposcopy provides an excellent view of the structure of the surface lining and makes it possible to detect suspicious areas from which samples can be taken. It is, or should be, the routine next step after a CERVICAL SMEAR TEST (*Pap test*) has shown some abnormality. The Royal College of Obstetricians and Gynaecologists has recommended that, ideally, no patient with surface cervical cancer (*intra-epithelial neoplasia*) should be treated without prior examination by colposcopy.

In addition to accurate diagnosis, colposcopy offers, in some cases, the advantage of local treatment under direct visual control. Lasers or other instruments can be used, and, in the hands of experienced gynaecologists, can offer great advantages over former methods. See also CONE BIOPSY.

Cone biopsy

The removal of a cone- or cylindrical-shaped segment of the neck of the UTERUS (*cervix*) which includes not only the lining but also some of the underlying tissue. Cone biopsy is done under general anaesthesia when a cervical smear test has suggested that an abnormality is present and microscopic examination of the cervix (*colposcopy*) does not fully demonstrate the abnormal area. It is used when there is suspicion of pre-malignancy. Bleeding is fairly common at the time of operation and between the 7th and 10th days afterwards. This is sometimes severe enough to require readmission to hospital and even, occasionally, blood transfusion. The scarring that follows this procedure may, rarely, reduce fertility and may lead to cervical incompetence, where the cervix is unable to remain properly closed and painless, spontaneous miscarriages result.

There is a trend to replace 'cold knife' cone biopsy with a method using a stainless steel wire loop heated by an electric current to remove the whole of the affected region of the cervix. This operation, called the loop electrosurgical excision procedure, takes about five minutes and may be done under local anaesthesia.

Cramps

A cramp is a minor disorder in which a single muscle, or a group of muscles, suddenly goes into a state of powerful sustained contraction. This causes severe pain which lasts until the contraction eases off. Cramp may be caused by excess salt loss from sweating and this type can be prevented by taking extra salt.

The common night cramps, which affect most people from time to time, usually involve the calf muscles. The cause has never been satisfactorily explained, but many people find that they can be prevented by taking a small dose of quinine.

Swimmers' cramp can affect the abdominal or limb muscles and sometimes leads to a panic reaction which only makes the situation worse. The best response is to tread water gently or float on the back until the spasm has passed and then to swim slowly, avoiding strenuous movements.

Creutzfeldt-Jakob disease

A few women have developed this disease after having chorionic gonadotrophin injections for infertility. Creutzfeldt-Jakob disease is a rapidly progressive disorder of the nervous system which affects middle-aged and elderly people causing death, usually within a year of onset. Sometimes called *suba-*

cute spongiform encephalopathy, it is an infection with a tiny protein particle called a *prion*. This is a very slow-acting agent with an incubation period of many years. It is unusually resistant to heat and to some other methods of sterilization, but can be destroyed by steam autoclaving.

The agent is known to have been transmitted by organ transplantation, neurosurgical operating instruments, and by human pituitary growth hormone injections, as well as the gonadotrophins. It is similar to the particle which causes a serious nervous system disease (*scrapie*) in sheep and *bovine spongiform encephalopathy* in cattle ('mad cow disease'). The brains of people with Creutzfeldt-Jakob disease show the same changes as are found in affected animals. The disease affects adults and is commonest in the late fifties. It takes many years to show itself, but once started, is fatal within a matter of months.

The first signs are usually irritability, fatigue, sleep disorders and neglect of personal hygiene. It soon becomes apparent that the affected person is suffering progressive dementia. Disturbance of any of the functions of the brain then become apparent. Increasing loss of memory and of intellectual function, loss of balance, paralysis, sensory loss, speech disorder, disorientation, tremor, twitching and other signs of progressive destruction of brain function occur, and the condition ends in death after a period of from three to 12 months.

There is no effective treatment. Fortunately, the chances of acquiring this dreadful disorder are very small. It affects only about one person per million of the population per year. There has been no evidence, to date, that it can be acquired by eating infected meat.

Cystitis

Cystitis is inflammation of the urinary bladder caused by infection. This is far commoner in women than in men mainly because of the shortness of the urine tube (*urethra*) from the bladder to the exterior. You may well be familiar with the symptoms. These are:

- unduly frequent desire to visit the toilet
- getting up at night to urinate
- frequent passage of small quantities of urine
- burning or 'scalding' pain on passing urine
- involuntary passage of a small squirt of urine on coughing or laughing (*stress incontinence*)

Sometimes you might even pass a little blood in the urine, making it look 'smoky'. Occasionally, in a severe attack, there may be fever, shivering, pain in the mid-back (*loins*) and generally feeling ill.

When urine from a person with cystitis is examined, bacteria are almost always found to be present. These are commonly *coliform* organisms of a kind that normally and harmlessly inhabit the bowel. However, cystitis may be due to other germs, including those acquired during sexual intercourse such as *Chlamydia* (see CHLAMYDIAL INFECTIONS), *Trichomonas* and THRUSH. If you have more than very occasional attacks of cystitis your doctor will probably arrange for you to be seen by a urological specialist to check whether there is anything else wrong with your waterworks.

Most cases of cystitis can be effectively treated with antibiotics or a mixture of a sulphonamide drug and a folic acid inhibitor (Septrin). This should be rapidly effective. If not, further investigation is called for in case the infection should be of wider extent or should be connected with some other bladder or kidney problem. In menopausal women, cystitis may respond better to oestrogens than to antibiotics. This is because after the menopause the shortage of oestrogens discourages the growth of vaginal lactobacilli. These organisms produce lactic acid and this keeps other germs away. They are thus necessary for a healthy vagina. When the lactobacilli are not present the vagina becomes colonized by bowel organisms, especially *E. coli.* These are the commonest cause of urinary infection.

A report in the prestigious *New England Journal of Medicine* in September 1993 showed that a simple vaginal cream containing oestrogen, applied nightly for two weeks and then twice a week for eight months virtually eliminated urinary infection. The vaginal organisms were restored to the normal lactobacilli in those who were using the cream.

Cystitis can often be avoided by a few simple measures. These are:

- taking plenty of fluids to 'flush out' the urinary system
- patient attempts to continue after urination seems complete
- urination after sexual intercourse
- avoidance of nylon underwear
- no vaginal deodorants

D

Depression

Depression is a mood of sustained sadness or unhappiness. Numerous studies have shown that it is twice as common in women as in men. The reason for this is unknown. There is an important difference between normal unhappiness – which we all experience at times as a reaction to misfortune or boredom – and genuine depressive illness. Clinical depression involves a degree of hopeless despondency, dejection, fear and irritability out of all proportion to any external cause. Often there is no apparent cause. Associated symptoms include:

- a general slowing down of body and mind
- slow speech
- poor concentration
- confusion
- self-reproach
- self-accusation
- loss of self-esteem
- restlessness and agitation
- insomnia, with early morning waking
- loss of interest in sex

It is essential to be aware that suicide is an ever-present risk in people who are clinically depressed. Depression is especially common in elderly people. The highest incidence of first attacks occurs between the ages of 50 and 60 in women.

Depression is usually precipitated by a seriously afflicting major life event, such as a bereavement, retirement or loss of status. Postmenopausal depression is often attributed to hormonal changes but there is no positive proof of this.

The causes of depression remain speculative and there are probably many. Often it seems to be the result of a damaging tendency to view oneself as being undesirable, worthless, unwanted and unloved. A depressed person often views the world as a hostile place in which failure and punishment are to be expected and suffering and deprivation inevitable. Women may be particularly vulnerable as their sexual activity and energy decline. The loss of the ability to have children, after the menopause, may add to the sense of uselessness.

It is very important to recognize true depression in yourself or in someone you know so that urgent treatment can be given. In view of the danger and distress, and since the condition can in most cases be relieved, no time should be lost in seeking medical attention. Many depressed people who could have been restored to a normal emotional and social life have committed suicide. Effective antidepressant drugs, such as the tricyclics and the monoamine oxidase inhibitors, are available. But you should appreciate that these drugs do not show their effect until about two weeks after the treatment is started.

Dermabrasion

The passage of the years detracts from the beauty and uniformity of young skin. Evenness of skin colouring is a feature of youth and this is gradually lost as clumps of skin pigment, sometimes quite large, appear. Smoothness of surface gives way, over the years, to the cumulative effect of pitting scars from acne, chickenpox, pimples, boils and various minor injuries. Other accumulated blemishes which further damage the appearance include widened skin pores and ugly enlarged surface blood vessels. Finally, warts, moles, cysts of various kinds, skin tags and general roughness, all add their toll, so that the youthful appearance fades further and further into the background.

So, is there anything you can do to improve the appearance of the ageing skin? One answer is sandpapering. This may sound improbable, not to say brutal, but it is, in fact, a well-established method that has been used by dermatologists and plastic surgeons for years. To make it sound more clinical, the surgeons call it dermabrasion. This method was first found useful for the treatment of the very disfiguring tattooing of skin that commonly occurs in road traffic accidents, when gravel is driven into the face, or in gunshot or fireworks injuries, when the skin may be tattooed with particles of gunpowder. The method was also tried and found effective in the treatment of facial scarring from severe adolescent acne and is now quite commonly used for this. Dermabrasion has been found useful in the management of other kinds of scarring as well as fine skin wrinkles.

Some form of anaesthesia is essential and this may take the form of local injections of anaesthetic drugs or a freezing spray. In both cases, you will probably also have some sedation, as the process, however carefully done, can hardly be described as pleasant. Sometimes dermabrasion is done under general anaesthesia. The equipment is not particularly critical and machines designed for fine woodwork, with cylindrical drums of sandpaper are quite suitable. Indeed, although manufacturers of surgical equipment sell dermabrasion instruments, some surgeons prefer to use model-makers' sanding machines as some of these are kinder to the skin than the powerful, high-speed surgical equipment. Various sizes of sandpaper cylinder are used, depending on the kind of area being treated – large drums for flat areas and small for confined spaces, such as the angle of the nose. Whatever kind of equipment is used, it must have all its exposed parts – and especially the sanding drum – completely sterilized.

Dermabrasion causes quite severe bleeding because the process removes the outer layer of the skin and exposes, and ruptures, the tiny tufts of blood vessels in the deeper layers. During the sanding, the area being treated is constantly flooded with sterile salty water (*saline*) to wash away the blood and allow the surgeon to see exactly the level being reached. If the sanding goes too deep it will remove so much skin that regeneration is impossible and severe scarring will result. One fairly small area is done at a time and, if local anaesthetic is being used, repeated injections or freezing will be required as each new area is treated.

The principle of dermabrasion is to achieve a smooth surface by sanding down any areas which are raised, even if the skin in these areas is normal. In this way, pits and depressions become relatively less deep and obvious. This process will, of course, make the skin thinner. Because a new outer layer (*epidermis*) forms over the thinned deeper layer (*dermis*), the latter remains thin. The new epidermis grows from epidermal cells lining the hair follicles and sweat glands. These extend deeply into the skin so, even if quite a lot is sanded away, the supply of epidermal cells will remain to bud out a new outer layer for the abraded skin. But if the sanding is carried so deep that all the hair and sweat tubes are destroyed, then both you and the surgeon are in trouble.

Once sanding is complete, the now raw and bleeding areas are covered with sterile dressings, such as vaseline gauze, and protected by wool and bandages. Dressings are usually left in place for several days and it may be several weeks before your skin fully recovers. Sometimes, abraded areas remain red for a very long time – even for many months – and are especially sensitive to direct or reflected sunlight. This can cause changes in colour (*pigmentation*) which may seriously detract from the good effect of the treatment. In sunny climates, this sensitivity to sunlight can be so serious that some surgeons will do this operation only in winter.

Dilatation and curettage

This simple and commonly performed gynaecological operation is usually done under general anaesthesia. The surgeon gradually enlarges the canal of the opening into the UTERUS (*cervix*) by pushing in a succession of ever-wider smooth metal rods, called dilators, until it is wide enough to admit a long instrument with a small spoon-shaped head called a curette. With this, the inside of the uterus is gently scraped, either to remove the lining in the hope of relieving abnormal menstrual bleeding, to remove any unwanted tissue or to get a specimen (*biopsy*) for examination.

After MISCARRIAGE, dilatation and curettage is often used to get rid of 'retained products of conception' – an embryo that has failed to survive but has not been spontaneously expelled. The procedure was once commonly used to cause abortion in early pregnancy, but this is now usually done by suction curettage, using a fine tube.

Down's syndrome

Formerly called 'mongolism', Down's syndrome is of special concern to women who become pregnant late in their reproductive phase of life. It is a major genetic disorder caused by the presence, in the maternal ovum or the fertilizing sperm, of an extra chromosome 21. Thus the affected ovum, or sperm, as the case may be, has 24 chromosomes instead of the normal 23, and every cell in the body of an individual with Down's syndrome has 47 chromosomes instead of the normal 46. In genetic terminology, it is, for this reason, known as *trisomy 21*.

The incidence of the condition varies markedly with the age of the parents at the time of conception, especially with the age of the mother. For young women, the incidence is about one in 2000. For mothers approaching menopausal age, the incidence is about one in 40. The overall incidence is about one in 700. In about a quarter of the cases, the extra chromosome comes from the father.

People with Down's syndrome have oval, down-sloping eyelid openings and a large, protruding tongue, which does not show the normal central furrow. Around the edge of the irises of the eyes, greyish-white spots are visible soon after birth, but disappear within the first year. The head is short and wide and flattened at the back and the ears are small. The nose is short and with a depressed bridge and the lips thick and everted. The hands are broad, with a single palmar crease, and short fingers, and the skin tends to be rough and dry. The stature is low and usually the genitalia remain infantile. There is slow physical development and the muscle power is weak. There is a wide gap between the first and second toes. Other congenital disorders, such as heart and inner ear defects, are common and there is a special susceptibility to leukaemia. There is always some degree of mental defect, but this need not be severe and many people with Down's syndrome are able to engage in simple employment.

Formerly, people with Down's syndrome seldom survived childhood and many died from infections. Today, those without major heart problems usually survive, but the processes of ageing appear to be speeded up and most die in their forties or fifties.

Dysphagia

Difficulty in swallowing. It is very common to have a feeling of a 'lump in the throat' and a sense of difficulty in swallowing. This is not real dysphagia and is fairly harmless. Dysphagia is an organic disorder and may be due to a number of causes. These include:

- actual obstruction from a foreign body in the gullet
- a tumour of the gullet
- obstruction from external pressure on the gullet
- obstruction from a mass or abnormally placed structure outside the gullet
- oesophageal or pharyngeal pouch, into which some of the food passes
- a localized muscular constriction ring in the gullet
- a neurological disorder affecting the muscular contractions that control swallowing

DYSPHAEIA

If you have dysphagia you need urgent investigation including a barium swallow X-ray. This may show a local narrowing, or a *filling defect*, suggesting a tumour. In nervous system disorders, such as achalasia, neither fluids nor solids can be swallowed, but in tumour, fluids will often pass freely. Never neglect suspected dysphagia.

E

Endometriosis

The lining of the UTERUS – a highly specialized, hormone-sensitive membrane – is called the endometrium. Surprisingly, uterus lining sometimes also occurs in other places. This is always abnormal and is called endometriosis. Abnormally-sited endometrium may occur in the FALLOPIAN TUBES, on the ovaries, within the wall of the uterus itself, anywhere in the pelvis, or even further afield as in the lining of the nose and the lungs. The trouble is that, wherever it may be, endometrial tissue responds to the hormones that control the menstrual cycle. It thus goes through the same sequence of changes that affects the uterus lining. Menstrual blood from the uterus endometrium escapes through the vagina, but blood produced at these abnormal sites cannot usually escape, so there is a build-up of local pressure, and pain occurs with each menstrual period.

Endometriosis of the ovary – one of the commoner sites – can eventually cause a large cyst to develop and when this is removed it is found to be full of a dark chocolate-coloured fluid. Up to half of all infertile women have endometriosis.

As you might expect, the symptoms of endometriosis disappear during pregnancy and after the menopause. So it is easy to keep them at bay by continuously taking oral contraceptives or any other treatment that suppresses the function of the ovaries. The only complete cure, however, is to have these abnormal deposits of endometrium removed by surgery.

Endometritis

The endometrium is the inner lining of the UTERUS. Part of it is shed during the menstrual period. Afterwards it thickens up again, becomes more glandular, and develops an increased blood supply so as to be in a suitable state for the implantation and nourishment of the fertilized ovum. Inflammation of the endometrium, as a result of infection, is called endometritis. The most severe form of this is puerperal endometritis which sometimes occurs following childbirth. Another term for this is puerperal sepsis, and, before antibiotics were developed, this was a common cause of death after delivery.

Endometritis is uncommon except after delivery or abortion because of the protection of the vaginal acidity (see CYSTITIS) and because menstrual shedding carries away infected material. Childbirth endometritis is easily treated with antibiotics. After the menopause, the barriers to womb infection are less. Menopausal endometritis features a vaginal discharge with pus and sometimes blood. These are also the signs of UTERUS CANCER, so it is imperative that they should be reported without delay. Treatment of menopausal endometritis is highly effective and may involve oestrogen therapy, minor surgery and sometimes removal of the uterus (HYSTERECTOMY).

Exophthalmos

Bulging out of the eyeballs is known as exophthalmos. The forward movement of the eyes forces the eyelids apart and causes a staring appearance. The condition is caused by an increase in the bulk of the fat and muscles behind the eye in the bony eye socket. This occurs most commonly as a result of a THYROID GLAND DISORDER. In this case the thyroid gland is affected by an immune system defect that also results in masses of antibodies and white cells (*lymphocytes*) accumulating in the fat and muscles behind the eyes. The main effect is in the six small muscles that move each eye, and the action of these is sometimes interfered with. Thyroid exophthalmos does not necessarily occur at the same time as the active thyroid disease. Eye protrusion may occur months or years after a thyroid upset. It may, rarely, even precede it.

If you have persistent and disfiguring exophthalmos and especially if there is any question of risk to your vision from pressure on the optic nerves or exposure of the corneas, you should be under the care of an ophthalmic consultant. The question of relieving the protrusion and the pressure by removing the bony floors of the eye sockets will have to be considered. There is also the possibility of reinforcing your eyelids with mersilene mesh implants.

Although thyroid problems are by far the commonest cause of exophthalmos, even if only one eye appears to be affected, protrusion of an eyeball may be caused by the presence of other material in the orbit, such as a tumour. Eye protrusion must always be taken seriously and reported without delay.

F

Fainting

Fainting is a temporary loss of consciousness due to a drop in the blood pressure so that the brain is deprived of an adequate supply of fuel (glucose) and oxygen. The drop in blood pressure results either from a reduction in the rate of pumping of blood by the heart or from a general widening of the arteries of the body.

Common faints usually occur from simultaneous slowing of the heart and widening of the arteries, often after you have been standing for a long time, especially in a hot environment. Such conditions impede the return of blood to the heart by the veins. A severe fright or shock may cause sudden slowing of the heart, by way of the nerves that control the heart rate. Fainting is also more likely when the volume of your blood is reduced as occurs in fluid loss from prolonged diarrhoea or excessive sweating. Low blood pressure is normally desirable, but an abnormally low degree, as in Addison's disease or from over-enthusiastic treatment for high blood pressure, can be dangerous. Fainting on taking exercise suggests heart disease.

In a faint, the vision becomes misty, the ears ring, the skin becomes pale and the pulse slow. The resultant fall is exactly what is required to restore the flow of blood to the brain, and this can be encouraged by raising the legs. The last thing a fainting person needs is to be made to sit up. Convulsions or even brain damage can result if a fainting person is unadvisedly kept upright.

Fallopian tubes

These remarkable organs are the open-ended tubes that con-
duct eggs (*ova*) from the ovaries to the UTERUS. The outer, open,
end of each fallopian tube has many tiny, muscular, finger-like
tentacles, poised above the ovary. The inner surface of these
tentacles is lined with a membrane bearing millions of fine
hairs called cilia which move, like a wind-blown field of long
grass, so as to waft anything small enough into the tube. At
the time the egg is released (*ovulation*), these fingers sweep
over the surface of the ovary, covering about two thirds of its
upper surface. There is also a suction effect tending to draw
material into the tube.

The ovum has to be fertilized in the fallopian tube if the
timing of the development that follows is to be correct for
implantation into the lining of the uterus. So the sperms have
to get into the tube either just before or during the transit of
the egg.

Obstruction of the fallopian tubes from inflammation from
any cause results in sterility. Partial obstruction may prevent a
fertilized ovum from passing on into the uterus. The result
may be a dangerous out-of-uterus (*ectopic*) pregnancy.

The fallopian tubes are often deliberately clamped or cut
as a means of permanent contraception.

Fatigue

Tiredness may be physical or mental. Genuine physical
fatigue is due to the accumulation in the muscles of the breakdown products of fuel consumption and energy production
(*metabolism*). Resting for a short period will allow time for the
normal blood flow through the muscles to 'wash out' these

metabolites. In most cases, physical fatigue has a major mental element, and in many cases purely mental fatigue masquerades as physical fatigue.

Mental fatigue has nothing to do with over-use of the mental faculties. It is the result of boredom, over-long concentration on a single task, anxiety, frustration, fear, or just general disinclination to perform a particular job of work. People lucky enough to find their intellectual work absorbing may feel tired at the end of a day, but there is no persistent fatigue and the work is anticipated with pleasure.

Food irradiation

If food is exposed to strong ionising radiation, such as gamma rays, any bacteria and insect pests in it will be killed, and unwanted natural changes in fruit and vegetables delayed or stopped. Irradiation does not eliminate existing toxins or viruses. If the food is tightly sealed in a container, such as a polythene bag, before it is irradiated, organisms present are destroyed and no new organisms can gain access. Food treated in this way will keep indefinitely.

Food irradiation by gamma rays does not induce radioactivity, and the effects are chemical only. The main effect is the production of highly reactive, short-lived substances called free radicals which cause cell death in living organisms. Food molecules are also affected and there may be changes in flavour and some loss of vitamins.

A committee of the World Health Organisation has expressed the view that irradiation of any food commodity, up to a dose of one million rads, would present no nutritional or bacteriological hazard to the consumer. Experts from WHO point out the benefits of irradiation – the destruction of disease germs, such as salmonella in poultry; and the prolongation of shelf-life which would increase the food supply. Food irradiation is employed in nearly 40 countries, including Britain.

G

Gallstones

Under the age of 40 gallstones are three times as common in women as in men. They are especially common if you are overweight. Gallstones are hard round, oval, or faceted masses of stone-like material occurring in the gall bladder or the bile duct. Most gallstones are about the size of a pea or a marble, but may be multiple and very small, like fine gravel, or so large that a single stone completely fills the gall bladder. Gallstones do not necessarily cause trouble; about 40% of people over 60 have them, usually without any indication of the fact.

Most gallstones are composed of cholesterol, chalk (calcium carbonate), calcium bilirubinate, or a mixture of these. They are more likely to occur if the composition of the bile is abnormal, if there is blockage of bile outflow or local infection, or if there is a family history of gallstones. Their presence leads to inflammation of the gall bladder (*cholecystitis*), and may block the bile duct leading to yellowing of the skin (*obstructive jaundice*) from damming-back of the bile into the blood. The passage of a gallstone down the bile duct into the duodenum is a very painful experience, known as biliary colic.

Treatment is by removal of the gall bladder (*cholecystectomy*) – done by 'keyhole' laparoscopic surgery through very small incisions, or by gallstone *lithotripsy* in which stones are shattered by concentrated sound waves.

Goitre

Goitre simply means any enlargement of the thyroid gland, from any cause. The thyroid is situated across the front of the neck just below the Adam's apple. This gland produces hormones containing iodine, and a small quantity of this is necessary in the diet. If the iodine supply is insufficient, the gland increases its activity, producing excess of the incomplete hormone, and swells up. Iodine deficiency is almost unknown in Britain, mainly because a small quantity is artificially added to table salt. Goitre was once an epidemic condition in parts of Europe.

Goitre also occurs in the condition of Graves' disease, in which the gland is overactive and there is enlargement accompanied by excessive production of thyroid hormones. This is often associated with the staring condition of EXOPHTHALMOS. Other conditions causing goitre include:

- HASHIMOTO'S THYROIDITIS, caused by antibodies to thyroid hormone
- sub-acute thyroiditis, which is probably a virus infection
- dyshormonogenesis, a genetic enzyme deficiency which interferes with normal thyroid hormone synthesis
- tumours of the thyroid gland

See also THYROID GLAND DISORDERS.

H

Hair excess

Excess facial hair is common in women and generally distressing. It may, ironically, be associated with thinning and greying of the scalp hair. Unnatural hairiness, of this kind, is called *hirsutism* and, if severe, it is usually regarded as a major aesthetic blemish. There is never any real problem unless the hair is visible because of its colour. Blonde or bleached facial hair is inconspicuous and generally unobjectionable.

Hair follicles are a normal feature of all skin areas except the palms of the hands and the soles of the feet. In theory, therefore, hair can grow almost anywhere on the surface of the body. Even the external skin of the nose contains hair follicles and quite luxuriant growth of hair occasionally occurs, especially in men. Whether these follicles remain dormant or spring into productive life, depends on a number of factors. The most important of these are hormonal and it is primarily the sex hormones that determine the normal variations in hairiness between men and women.

Hirsutism in women does not, however, necessarily indicate that something has gone wrong with the sex hormones. In most cases there is no medical abnormality at all and the hairiness is either hereditary, or ethnic, or just plain bad luck. If the hirsutism is severe, however, medical investigation is certainly a good idea, because a number of important conditions can cause it. Perhaps the most significant is an excess of male sex hormone caused by hormone-secreting tumours of the ovaries or the adrenal glands. This would require urgent treatment.

Hirsutism may also be due to various genetic conditions. In rare cases, chromosomal examination shows the person concerned to be of the opposite sex to that assumed. Medical treatment can cause hirsutism, especially treatment with steroids, phenytoin (used for epilepsy or trigeminal neuralgia) and streptomycin. These last two drugs interfere with the excretion of steroids by the kidneys, so that they accumulate in the bloodstream, and this may be the way in which they promote hirsutism. Some races are ethnically predisposed to hairiness and there is a genetic condition in which hair follicles become sensitized to the low levels of male sex hormone normally present in the bloodstream of women.

If, as is often the case, these factors cannot be controlled, we are left with the problem of what to do about the unwanted hair. Hairs plucked from the follicles, whether individually or *en masse* by waxing, grow to full length again in four to six weeks and the process must be regularly repeated. Shaving is easier and less painful and is almost as effective as plucking. Contrary to widespread belief, shaving does not cause hairs to become thicker and stronger. The fallacy has arisen because of what happens to the hair of adolescent males after they start shaving. But it is not the shaving that causes the toughening of the beard – simply the hormone-induced heavier growth of hair. Of course, short-shaved hairs will always feel more bristly than long hairs, and this, too, adds to the illusion.

Depilatories

These are preparations for removing hair. Various chemicals, such as barium sulphide or thioglycolic acid salts, can soften and dissolve hairs, so that they can be wiped off, but those that are safe do not affect the follicles, and the hair grows again. Any chemical capable of softening hair is bound to be hard on the skin, so use them with care. Avoid those that cause any obvious skin inflammation.

Electrolysis

This is a fancy name for a very simple process which removes hair permanently, but one which requires skill – and good eyesight. The word *electrolysis* means the breaking down of water into its two component gases – oxygen and hydrogen – by the passage of an electric current. It is not, however, the electrolysis that destroys the hair follicle, but rather the burning effect of the high current density at the point of application. The method is simple. You are connected to a source of electricity at low voltage via a broad pad of saline-moistened lint on which is pressed, by means of a strap, one of the metal electrodes. The other electrode is a very fine needle and when this touches your skin and the switch is closed, the circuit is completed.

The needle is pushed carefully into the hair follicle and this is most easily done using a low-powered operating microscope. When the current is turned on, the follicle is literally fried up and turns into a small scar. The current passing is registered on a milliammeter and is checked regularly. Although you may feel a strong sensation, the instrument is incapable of providing a dangerous current. The operator can tell if the application has been effective by the appearance of a small foam of gas bubbles around the shaft of the hair and by its loosening, so that it can be lifted out without the need for any force.

As only one hair can be dealt with at a time, this is clearly a tedious, time-consuming and uncomfortable business. When the foot-switch is pressed to turn on the current, you will be keenly aware of a tiny electric shock and, of course, this will be repeated many times. The operator must try to keep the current within a reasonable range, not only to avoid discomfort, but also to avoid unnecessary scarring of the skin, and this is not always easy. Sometimes a local anaesthetic is used, but this increases the risk of scarring as you will not be aware of, or object to, excessive current.

The results depend largely on the skill of the operator in placing the needle accurately and in controlling the current. If hairs are simply plucked out after inaccurate applications, they will, of course, grow again and you will have wasted your money.

Electrolysis is not all it is cracked up to be and has been condemned by some surgeons. Many dermatologists, having considered all the available methods for the removal of unwanted hair in women, have concluded that shaving (either with a good electric shaver or one of today's sophisticated double-blade razors) is probably best.

Skin grafting

This has a very small part to play in the management of hirsutism, which is usually too widespread to make grafting feasible. Moreover, it may be very difficult to find a donor area that is not, itself, hairy. Grafting is justified in those rare cases in which the excess hair is confined to a small, localized patch. Hairy moles can easily be removed and the skin can usually be closed directly without grafting. But if they are large, a free skin graft can be taken, perhaps from behind the ear, to cover the deficit.

The commonly affected parts in female hirsutism – the moustache and beard areas – are not at all suitable for grafting. If you were able to persuade a surgeon to do this, you would probably end up looking worse than you started. It is very difficult to match the texture and colour of facial skin with skin taken from any other part of the body, and such grafts, done to cover burned or injured areas, are apt to be rather conspicuous. You will be much better to rely on bleaching and shaving.

Hashimoto's thyroiditis

This is a swelling of the thyroid gland, a form of GOITRE, that causes an ache in the neck and sometimes difficulty in swallowing. This form of thyroid gland disorder is commonest in middle-aged women and is due to the formation of antibodies to the protein from which the hormones are synthesized. These antibodies can be found in the blood, often in large quantities, and they return to the gland and attack it as if it were foreign tissue, causing inflammation and damage.

The condition responds well to administration of thyroid hormone (*thyroxine*) and this is continued indefinitely, as the gland will eventually become underactive. Steroids may also be required.

Heartburn

A burning or aching sensation felt behind the lower part of the breastbone when a short length of the gullet (*oesophagus*) squeezes itself (spasm) or when acid from the stomach is forced up into the gullet. Heartburn is commonest after meals, especially if you have been indulging injudiciously in fatty foods. It is also worse you are lying down and acid can more easily get into the gullet. For the same reason, heartburn is common in pregnancy. It is often associated with 'waterbrash' in which bitter-tasting stomach contents come right up into your mouth.

A common cause of heartburn is hiatus hernia in which part of the stomach pushes upwards, through the normal opening in the diaphragm, into the chest.

Heartburn can be prevented by eating more wisely, more slowly and more abstemiously. See that you get proper medical attention for duodenal (*peptic*) ulceration. There have been important recent advances in the management of these conditions.

Hip replacement

Because the high incidence of osteoporosis in women after the menopause leads to many fractures of the neck of the thigh bone, this operation has become one of the most commonly performed on women. Tens of thousands of hip replacement operations are done every year in Britain. The operation is highly successful as both the natural socket (*acetabulum*) and the natural ball, the head of the thigh bone (*femur*), are replaced. In the operation, the joint, which has been grossly damaged by loss of its blood supply or by arthritis, is completely removed. It is replaced by a plastic socket fitted into the hollow in the pelvis, and a short, angled metal shaft, which is force down into the hollow of the thigh bone, and which has on its upper end a smooth ball to fit into the socket.

The hip replacement operation is so common that you may think of it as a routine and simple procedure. This is not so. Hip replacement is major surgery, calling for great skill and substantial surgical resources. It is expensive and time-consuming. But the results are so good that, as in the case of intra-ocular lens implants for cataract, the time, trouble and cost are irrelevant.

Complications do occur, the most important being infection and loosening of the shaft of the prosthesis in the hollow of the thigh bone. The infection rate, in spite of the most elaborate precautions, is usually at least 1%. Loosening, especially after a number of years, has been a major problem and has, so far, defied the ingenuity of technology. Special bone glues are commonly used but problems of differences of elasticity between cement and bone still have to be resolved. Re-operation may be necessary in such cases. Infection may call for surgical draining and prolonged antibiotic treatment.

Holistic medicine

The holistic movement within medicine arose as a reaction against the way technology tends to exclude human factors and relationships. Critics rightly point out that a system which manages patients in a depersonalized way, treating them as machines to be modified by drugs, is neither optimum nor particularly effective. They suggest that the doctor's function is not simply to treat a diseased organ but also to consider the patient as a whole person in his or her cultural and environmental context, with feelings, attitudes, fears and prejudices.

This is especially important of male doctors' attitudes to female patients, for it is not always easy for male doctors to envisage the special feelings of vulnerability suffered by many women when ill. For many reasons – overwork, undue preoccupation with technology, emotional poverty, fear of improper involvement – true empathy with patients is rare. This is particularly unfortunate in an age when women, while better informed than ever before of the harm that may befall them, may, at the same time, feel inadequate to enquire into, and insist on having, all the resources of modern medicine.

One hundred years ago, when doctors had at their command only a fraction of the present resources, their concern and anxiety for their patients were much more obvious than today. As a result, the reputation of the profession stood much higher than it does now. You should not infer from this, however, that doctors care less about you than they used to.

Holistic medicine has always, throughout the ages, been practised by the best of the profession; but it is right and proper, in this mechanistic age, that we should all be reminded of what this means, and of how important it is.

Hormone replacement therapy (HRT)

Sex hormones (synthetic oestrogens) are available to alleviate immediate menopausal symptoms such as hot flushes, depression, irritability, sweating and insomnia. Doctors are generally agreed that such treatment is useful in the short term. There is less complete agreement about the longer term use of hormone replacement therapy (HRT) to treat the OSTEOPOROSIS which is so common after the menopause, and the tendency to drying up, shrinkage and infection of the vagina, which sometimes affects postmenopausal women. The results of many recent studies have, however, led to a progressive swing in favour of it. Decisions on HRT are, however, for you to make, and you should be in full possession of the facts.

Osteoporosis is often a serious matter, causing severe bowing of the spine or leading to fracture of the hip bone on minor physical stress (see HIP REPLACEMENT). Some women lose bone strength rapidly and these are especially at risk of the worst effects, while others seem to lose bone mass only at about the normal rate associated with ageing in both sexes. Osteoporosis causes hip fractures in about a quarter of elderly women. Women who have an early menopause are especially at risk, and HRT can largely eliminate the additional risk women suffer after the menopause. It is established that the chances of bone fracture can be halved by long-term HRT.

You should, however, understand the risks. Oestrogens alone, increase the risk of BREAST CANCER and UTERUS CANCER. At least 10 reliable studies have shown an increased occurrence of breast cancer after five years of HRT. It is difficult to get consistent figures for the increase in the risk. Of nearly 2,000 women in Kentucky who were given oestrogens after the menopause, and followed up for an average of twelve years, 49 developed breast cancer. The expected figure, for the general population, was 39, so 10 extra cases in 2,000 were, apparently, caused by the treatment. The worst reported series found an average increase to 1.6 women for every woman not on HRT. The important thing is that almost all series show that although there is an increased incidence of breast cancer, there is a *decreased mortality from breast cancer*, with greatly increased survival, among women on HRT. This important fact has led some authorities to state that fear of breast cancer is no reason to avoid HRT.

There is another reason for increased survival in women on HRT. Until the menopause, women are much less liable to heart attacks than men. This is because female sex hormones are protective against the arterial disease atherosclerosis that causes the trouble. After the menopause, the incidence of atherosclerosis rises steeply in women. HRT allows this protective effect to continue, and this has been borne out in a number of studies.

Oestrogen alone increases the risk of cancer of the lining of the uterus (*endometrial cancer*). Before the menopause, natural oestrogens are balanced by progesterone. Studies have now clearly shown that oestrogen replacement therapy combined with progesterone reduces this risk to that of the general population. There are, however, a number of snags. You are not likely to be very keen to start menstruating again. Regular bleeding also makes it more difficult to detect early bleeding from a cancer. If there is any question of abnormal or irregular bleeding you will need a DILATATION AND CURETTAGE to be sure you are safe.

Unfortunately, also, the mood improvement enjoyed from oestrogens is countered by progesterone, which may bring on a pattern identical to that of the premenstrual syndrome. If you have had your uterus removed, there is, of course, no problem and you do not need progesterone. Indeed women who have had a HYSTERECTOMY are fortunate in being able to have all the benefits of HRT with few disadvantages.

HRT causes no increase in cancer of the cervix, ovary or vulva, and worry about an increase in other cancers is unjustified. The overall mortality from all cancers in postmenopausal women taking HRT is lower than in postmenopausal women not taking HRT. Hormone replacement therapy does not increase the risk of high blood pressure, deep vein thrombosis or blood clots travelling to the lungs (*pulmonary embolism*). It reduces the risk of heart attacks and strokes.

The effects of HRT depend to some extent on the way it is given, and HRT by mouth is not necessarily best. Everything absorbed from the intestine goes straight to the liver and oestrogens are changed in the liver into a less active form. This may be sufficient to prevent the hormone from exercising its full bone-protective function. If you take your HRT by way of the skin this does not happen, as the hormone passes directly into the general circulation. Skin patches do cause their own problems, however. They can cause skin reactions and can get detached. Direct pellet implants under the skin are more reliable. This requires a minor operation under local anaesthesia every six months or so. New synthetic drugs with oestrogen action and fewer side-effects are being developed. One of these, now available, is Livial (tibolone).

Most doctors, although thoroughly familiar with the distressing effects of oestrogen deprivation in women, are surprisingly uninterested in long-term HRT for postmenopausal women. Only about 9% of postmenopausal women in London receive HRT for more than three years. Even women who have had their ovaries removed before the age of 30 and who are at high risk from osteoporosis as well as increased risk of heart attacks and strokes, are not offered HRT early enough to prevent these diseases. Those who know most about the matter, however, are all strongly in favour of HRT. One respectable authority, writing in the *Journal of the Royal Society of Medicine* in 1992 stated: 'Oestrogen replacement therapy is probably the most important advance in preventive medicine in the Western world for the last half century.'

Hymen

This is the thin, perforated membrane that stretches over the opening of the vagina in young women and usually tears spontaneously before puberty. Sometimes the hymen is exceptionally thick, or it may even completely close off the vaginal orifice. This rare event is called imperforate hymen and requires surgical incision to allow menstrual fluid to escape. Quite often there is some hymen left at the time of the first full act of sexual intercourse. In such a case this generally gets torn and there may be a little bleeding. The notion that all virgins bleed on 'defloration' is wrong.

Hyperhidrosis

This is the medical term for excessive sweating due to overactivity of the sweat glands. This may occur all over the skin, or may be confined to certain areas, such as the palms of the hands, the armpits, the groins and the feet. In severe cases, areas of the skin may become soggy and softened from being constantly wet. Hyperhidrosis often causes strong BODY ODOUR, as a result of bacterial breakdown of the sweat and the surface cells of the skin. This is called bromhidrosis.

The condition is usually just a variant of the normal, but may be caused by thyroid gland overactivity, fever and, rarely, a disease of the nervous system. In some cases, local hyperhidrosis is due to stress reactions or other psychological causes. It can be treated by local applications to reduce the activity of the sweat glands, or even, in extreme cases, by the surgical removal of the most active groups of glands. Many people just naturally sweat a lot, and require more than average body bathing and clothes washing. Emotional sweating usually resolves with time.

Hyperventilation

Very deep or rapid breathing occurs normally as a feature of violent exercise. The term is, however, more often applied to a degree of deep breathing inappropriate to the oxygen needs of the body. In such cases there is excessive and abnormal loss of carbon dioxide from the blood. The result is a reduction in blood acidity. This, in turn, affects the levels of calcium in the blood, which brings about various changes in the conductance of nerves so that certain muscle groups, such as those of the forearms and calves, may go into intense spasm causing the wrists to bend and the ankles to extend.

Hyperventilation is a common panic reaction and is associated with an alarming feeling of 'not getting enough air'. It also sometimes occurs in people who feel that they are not getting enough attention. In this, the activity is usually highly successful, but is not entirely without danger. The right response is to try to persuade the affected person to re-breathe for a few minutes into a small paper or plastic bag. If this is done, carbon dioxide is returned to the blood, the blood changes are soon reversed and the drama is over.

In very rare cases, hyperventilation can be an effect of organic disease such as brain damage from infection or injury, poisoning, fever or thyroid gland overactivity. In all of these, however, there are other obvious signs of illness.

Hysterectomy

Hysterectomy means surgical removal of the UTERUS. This can be done through the vagina, or, more easily, through an incision in the front wall of the abdomen. Hysterectomy is done for a variety of reasons including:

- cancer of the UTERUS
- ENDOMETRIOSIS
- large fibroids
- severely excessive menstruation (*menorrhagia*)
- excessive menstrual pain
- occasionally for sterilization

For various reasons, hysterectomy has been a very commonly performed operation in the past, especially in the USA. An estimated half a million women have a hysterectomy every year. Not so long ago about a quarter of all American women over 50 had had the operation. In Britain, hysterectomy is performed less often.

The operation may be 'subtotal', in which the body of the uterus is removed but the neck (*cervix*) is left, or total, in which the upper part of the vagina is cut around and has to be sewn closed. The latter is now the more usual procedure. A Wertheim's hysterectomy, for cancer, involves removal of the uterus, fallopian tubes and ovaries, the upper third of the vagina and all the lymph nodes in the region.

In vaginal total hysterectomy, the cervix is grasped in toothed forceps and the uterus pulled down so that the vagina is turned partly inside out. A cut is then made around the cervix and down the front wall of the vagina. This allows the surgeon to get access to the attachments of the uterus to the side walls of the pelvis, so that these can be cut and the uterus removed. The floor of the pelvis is then strengthened by stitching muscles together and the opening in the vagina is stitched closed. This approach avoids a visible scar on the abdomen, but has the disadvantage that the vaginal scars are more extensive.

After abdominal hysterectomy the vaginal scar is confined to the upper end, which becomes a blind-ended tube. No ill effects arise as a result of the slight shortening of the vagina, as this structure is very elastic and stretches easily. Sexual intercourse is best avoided for about six weeks after a hysterectomy. Any subsequent problems with sexual intercourse are unlikely to be caused by shortening or scarring, but may arise from hormone deficiency, if the ovaries have been removed.

Many women who have had a hysterectomy feel less worthy, or in some way damaged and less attractive to their partners, and it is not uncommon for women deliberately to avoid sex. Loss of libido is, of course, commonly associated with the kind of serious illnesses that have required hysterectomy. Sexual interest will, hopefully, return with recovery. Sexual problems following hysterectomy are essentially psychological and may be difficult to overcome. Psychotherapy, and especially behaviour therapy with a definite program of deliberate sexual activity, have been found to be the most effective approach. The awareness of no longer being able to bear children can add to psychological difficulties.

I

Incontinence

Urinary incontinence in women is far commoner than is generally supposed. Up to half of all women have experienced it and about 7% suffer regularly from this embarrassing and distressing complaint. No one wants to talk about urinary incontinence – the involuntary and undesired passing of urine. As a result, thousands of women suffer in silence. Only a third of them receive medical care or help from the social services. Incontinence is commoner in the elderly than in the young, but many young women suffer from it. Older people are more often affected mainly because the strength of the circular muscles (*sphincters*), which keep the urine tube (*urethra*) closed until voluntarily relaxed, weaken progressively with age. In addition, older women are more likely to have suffered injury to the muscles of the floor of the pelvis in childbirth. Infection of the urinary tract, also common in the elderly, is another contributory cause. There are three main types of incontinence.

Stress incontinence

This very common form features the escape of a small amount of urine when pressure is involuntarily applied to the bladder during coughing, sneezing, laughing, weight-bearing or strenuous activity. It especially affects women who have had babies and whose urethral sphincters have been stretched. It is also commonly caused by weakening of pelvic muscles in childbirth, urinary tract infections, bladder stones or by a downward displacement (*prolapse*) of the UTERUS or vagina.

Urge incontinence
More distressing is urge incontinence, in which, at a certain level of bladder internal pressure, the strong urge to pass urine is followed by involuntary and uncontrollable bladder contraction, so that it empties completely. Urge incontinence can happen at any time and during any activity, or even at rest, and is often triggered by a sudden change of position.

Irritable bladder
This is a condition in which, for various reasons, the bladder muscle contracts intermittently, pushing out a little urine into the beginning of the urethra. As soon as this happens, the pressure of urine at this point in the urethra, causes an intense desire to relax the sphincter and pass urine. This is another cause of urge incontinence.

Treating incontinence
The first thing the doctors have to do is to find the cause. If there is bladder infection, this must be treated. Examination of a sample of urine is necessary and often reveals the cause. X-rays, including special methods using a dye that is rapidly excreted and shows up on the plate (*intravenous urography*) will detect obstructions, stones and structural abnormalities. Ultrasound scanning can also be used. The muscle and nerve function of the bladder can be tested by measuring the internal bladder pressure. Sometimes it is necessary to examine the inside of the bladder directly by passing a narrow viewing tube called a cystoscope along the urethra. This may reveal stones, polyps or tumours.

Weak pelvic muscles can be strengthened by pelvic floor exercises and these can help to restore sphincter function. Occasionally, surgical tightening of the muscles may be needed. In extreme cases, an artificial sphincter, that can be controlled from the outside, can be implanted around the urethra. Rarely, the solution may be to bypass the bladder altogether.

While, obviously, treatment and cure is best, many affected women prefer to use special incontinence clothing or urine collecting devices. Self-catheterization, to keep the bladder empty by draining it through a tube, is a possibility in some cases. For irritable bladder, drugs are sometimes used to relax the bladder muscle.

Faecal incontinence

Ironically, inability to retain faeces in the rectum is usually caused by chronic constipation. The faeces become hardened and cause irritation to the rectal lining with increased peristaltic effort. As a result, fluid and small faeces are involuntarily forced out. Proper management of the constipation – high fibre intake, suppositories of glycerol or mild laxative drugs, or softening and bulking agents – will cure this type of incontinence. Less commonly, faecal incontinence may result from:

- organic disorder – injury the anal canal muscles from a tear during childbirth
- neurological problems such as paraplegia or multiple sclerosis
- organic brain syndrome
- dementia

In some of these cases, faecal incontinence can be avoided by the use of regular enemas to keep the rectum empty.

Infertility

If everything is working properly in both you and your partner and you are having sex at least twice a week, you can expect to get pregnant within a few months of starting to try for a baby. If nothing happens for a year, you will have to assume that there is some degree of infertility. About 10% of couples have this problem. Fertility is not much affected by your general health or nutrition. But if you diet too strictly your periods may stop and there will be no ovulation. Very enthusiastic athletic training may also prevent ovulation. The same goes for underactivity of the thyroid gland and badly controlled diabetes.

A review of the menstrual cycle and ovulation would be helpful at this point. Between the start of the bleeding in one cycle and the start of the next, the time, on average, is 28 days. But periods may be as short as 21 days, or, in extreme cases, as long as 60. This cycle is controlled by hormones from the pituitary gland which is an outgrowth of the brain. The follicle-stimulating hormone (FSH) from the pituitary gland acts on one of the ovaries to cause a collection of cells, containing an egg, to develop. This nest of cells is called a Graafian follicle. During the first half of the menstrual cycle the Graafian follicle produces increasing amounts of oestrogen hormone. This hormone causes thickening of the lining of the UTERUS and an increase in its blood vessels and mucus glands.

In the middle of the cycle the egg is released from the follicle in the ovary. This is called ovulation. But the follicle has not yet fully served its purpose. The cells of the empty follicle develop into a mass called the *corpus luteum*, which begins to secrete progesterone, a hormone necessary to maintain the lining of the uterus so that it is suitable to support a pregnancy. If the ovum is not fertilized, the corpus luteum degenerates and progesterone production drops off. This causes the lining of the uterus to be discarded as menstruation, about 14 days after the time of ovulation. The vaginal blood loss that occurs when the body's level of progesterone or oestrogen hormones drops suddenly is called withdrawal bleeding. Normal menstruation is preceded by withdrawal of both oestrogen and progesterone. Similar withdrawal bleeding occurs at the end of each cycle of combined oral contraceptive pills, but is usually shorter and lighter. It is the withdrawal of progesterone that produces the blood loss.

The release of an egg from the ovary is called ovulation. A released egg is swept into the FALLOPIAN TUBE and carried along towards the uterus. While in the tube, it may be met by sperms (*spermatozoa*). If not, the egg is simply discarded during the next menstruation. If pregnancy does occur, the placenta, almost as soon as it is established, begins to secrete a hormone that keeps the corpus luteum going so that the supply of progesterone is maintained for the first three months or so. After that, the placenta takes over the oestrogen and progesterone production, so that no further ovulation or menstruation occurs during the remainder of the pregnancy.

Even if you are ovulating, this may happen infrequently enough to prevent conception by sheer accident of timing. Irregular, unpredictable and infrequent egg production will, of course, reduce the chance of the egg and sperm meeting. Various tests can be done to check whether you are ovulating.

If not, you can have hormones or other drugs to stimulate ovulation, or prevent it from being inhibited. The main drugs used are anti-oestrogens such as clomiphene or TAMOXIFEN. Some of these drugs are so effective that infertile couples surprise everyone by producing twins. Another method is to give 'pulsed' doses of a hormone called gonadotrophin releasing hormone. This prompts the pituitary gland to produce the hormones that cause ovulation. Other drugs used are human menopausal gonadotrophin (HMG) and human chorionic gonadotrophin (HCG). These can cause multiple pregnancies unless the hormone levels are carefully monitored.

Tests for ovulation include the measurement of blood progesterone levels, which rise in the second half of the cycle, as well as examination of the mucus in the cervix which changes at ovulation. Sometimes the pain on ovulation ('*mittelschmerz*') is severe and positive enough to indicate what is happening. In general, regular menstruation suggests that ovulation is occurring.

Infertility is commonly caused by mechanical blockage of the fallopian tubes, so that the egg and sperms are kept apart. This is almost always the result of infection. This is commonly the result of a sexually transmitted disease but may also follow the normal delivery of a baby or an abortion. Pelvic infection can also result from a burst inflamed appendix or tuberculosis. The state of your fallopian tubes can be investigated by injecting a harmless dye through the cervix. If the tubes are clear the dye will pass through the outer open ends of the tubes and can be observed through a narrow optical instrument called a laparoscope. This is passed through the abdominal wall. Laparoscopy also lets the doctor inspect your tubes for visible abnormalities and your ovaries for the presence of a Graafian follicles or a corpus luteum. Blocked tubes can sometimes be reopened, but this is difficult.

Before you are put through all this, however, your partner must have a sperm count. This is easy and quick and is always done before the female investigation. Male infertility is almost entirely a question of the sperm count and whether the sperms are normal and sufficiently active. If there are no sperms in the semen there is no possibility of fertilization. The masturbation specimen should have a volume of 2–6 ml and should contain 20,000,000 sperms per ml. More than 40% of these should be energetically motile and fewer than 30% should have an abnormal appearance. It's worth remembering that long-term alcohol excess causes a low sperm count and that this usually comes back to normal if drinking is moderated. In some cases of low sperm count, treatment with synthetic male sex hormones is effective.

Artificial insemination

If the problem is in the sperms or is due to impotence or other failure of normal sexual intercourse, you might want to consider artificial insemination. This is very simple and you can easily do it yourself, or get your partner to do it. A quantity of fresh seminal fluid donated by your husband (AIH), your partner (AIP) or by an anonymous donor (AID) is sucked up into a narrow syringe or pipette and injected high into the vagina or even into the mucus in the cervix. Impotent husbands can usually provide semen by masturbation. Of course, you have to time the procedure to coincide with the period in the menstrual cycle when ovulation is most likely. This usually occurs 14 days before the next period would have started. So you can estimate the best time on the basis of your usual cycle. Assuming no other reasons for infertility, the success rate is as high as in couples without such specific problems.

Sperm donation

Since the 1940s, human seminal fluid has been preserved, for indefinite periods, frozen in a glycerol cryoprotectant. Sperm is stored in phials, or plastic straws, in liquid nitrogen sperm banks. Sperm donation is used in cases of male sterility, dominant genetic disease and recessive disease where both husband and wife carry the gene. Banked semen is simply thawed, sucked up into a fine syringe and injected. Fresh semen can also be used, and this is produced, by masturbation, within a few hours of use. The insemination may be done in a doctor's surgery, in a sperm centre, or in your own home.

Unless the husband's or partner's semen is used, donors are nearly always anonymous. In Britain, many of them are medical students. Whoever is the donor, elaborate precautions are taken to ensure complete screening against AIDS and hepatitis B. The largest sperm bank is the Centre d'Etude et de Conservation du Sperm Humain (CECOS) in France. There, donors are asked to give one, two or three ejaculates a week for a month and then never again. The plastic straws in which the semen is stored each contain enough for one insemination, and a liberal supplier can fill over two hundred of these straws.

A child born from fertilization by donated sperm is deemed, by a legal presumption, to be the legitimate child of the husband. Since the procedure involves no sexual act, it is not generally considered adultery, but the Roman Catholic church has reservations.

In vitro fertilization

In vitro just means 'in glass' and refers to a procedure in which living eggs are taken from a woman's ovary, fertilized by sperm in a sterile glass dish, and replaced in the uterus. There are no end of difficulties and the success rate is not high – no more than 10%. Ovulation is stimulated with drugs or hormones and the growth of the Graafian follicles checked by ultrasound. When a follicle reaches a size of about 1.5 mm, a dose of follicle-stimulating hormone is given to prompt the release of eggs. These, usually up to 10, are collected using a fine needle guided by the ultrasound image. The eggs are kept at body temperature in a suitable culture medium for four to six hours and then the sperm are added. The fertilized eggs are kept in the medium for about two days, and then two or three of them are placed in the uterus through a fine tube. Spare embryos can be frozen and kept for a later attempt if the first is not successful.

At present, in spite of remarkable advances, in vitro fertilization is the least successful way of dealing with infertility. In addition to the low success rate, babies born in this way have a somewhat higher chance of problems such as prematurity and developmental abnormalities. Tragically, as many as 50% of pregnancies brought about in this way do not result in an uncomplicated live birth. You should really consider it a last resort.

Gamete intrafallopian transfer (GIFT) is a method in which eggs are collected as described and then injected, along with some sperm, into the open end of one of the fallopian tubes. This is done through a laparoscope (see PELVIC EXAMINATION). This method is often effective in cases of unexplained infertility.

Irritable bowel syndrome

This is the current term for a condition that has been known to doctors for many years under various names such as *spastic colon*, *nervous diarrhoea* or *idiopathic diarrhoea*. It is a persistent disorder for which no organic cause can be found. It features recurrent abdominal pain and intermittent diarrhoea often alternating with constipation.

This distressing disorder most commonly affects women between 20 and 40. The pain is usually felt in one of the four corners of the abdomen, is sometimes brought on by eating, and is often relieved by going to the toilet. The stools are usually ribbon-like or pellet-like and may contain mucus. Often, soon after a meal, there is extreme and embarrassing urgency to empty the bowels. There may be loud abdominal rumblings and squeaking (*borborygmi*), excessive gas production (*flatus*), headache, tiredness and nausea. Sometimes there is a sense of incomplete emptying after defaecation.

The condition tends to affect anxious, tense, intelligent, conscientious women, especially those who worry unduly about personal, family and financial matters. There may be an underlying fear of cancer. Full investigation, including barium meal X-ray, shows no objective abnormality, but, on examination, the colon is seen to be in a state of unusual activity, contracting and relaxing in an abnormally rapid manner.

A diet high in roughage is helpful in regulating the bowel

action, and there are several drugs effective in quieting down the excessive bowel activity and relieving the pain. Drugs can be carried and taken in anticipation of events which might provoke an acute attack.

K

Kleptomania

This is a rare condition in which the sufferer repeatedly fails to resist the impulse to steal things she doesn't need or particularly want. The objects are usually taken from a shop. Kleptomaniacs are usually well able to pay for the things they steal and the motive is not the same as that of the thief.

The act is not usually pre-planned and the object is the theft itself rather than the acquisition. As in other impulse disorders, there is a rising sense of tension focused on the actual shoplifting, with a relief of tension and a sense of elation when the act is accomplished. This may, however, be followed by strong guilt feelings and intense fear of discovery. The stolen objects are usually given away or otherwise disposed of.

Although kleptomania is often put forward as a defence against a charge of theft, it is in fact very uncommon. Less than 5% of people arrested for shoplifting are found to respond to questioning in a manner consistent with the diagnosis of kleptomania. The condition is associated with stress, such as bereavement or separation, and kleptomaniacs also tend to suffer from persistent depression and ANOREXIA NERVOSA. Kleptomaniacs often seem to have given no thought to the probable consequences of their actions and some appear outraged if they are arrested. They have been described as people who feel wronged and thus entitled to steal.

The cause is unknown, but some very odd explanations have been proposed by psychoanalysts. These include the suggestion that:

- all stealing is rooted in the essential oneness between mother and child (Anna Freud)
- it represents a search for a penis
- it is a means of seeking punishment
- it is an excitement, enjoyed as a substitute for sexual intercourse

L

Labia

The labia (singular *labium*) are the four elongated lips that surround the entrance to your vagina and the external opening of the urine tube (*urethra*). The inner of the two pairs, the *labia minora*, are narrow, wrinkled and red and vary in depth in different women. Each one forks, at the front, to form a hood over the front of the head of the clitoris. The outer pair, the *labia majora*, are long, well padded folds, containing muscle and fatty tissue, and are covered with hair. At the front, they join in the lower part of the pubic mound (*mons veneris*). As they run back between the thighs, they become more prominent. Behind, they join together a few centimetres in front of the anus. They are normally closed and conceal the rest of the genitalia.

There is not much to go wrong with the labia apart from inflammation from THRUSH (*vulvitis*) or herpes, genital warts or the effects of sexually transmitted diseases. Occasionally a large lip may be affected by an abscess in one of the Bartholin's glands which lie between the back part of the vaginal opening and the labia minora.

Laparoscopy

See PELVIC EXAMINATION.

Lumpectomy

An operation for breast cancer in which no attempt is made to remove more than the obvious lump. Supplementary treatment with radiation or chemotherapy is then given. Lumpectomy is also used for benign lumps. See BREAST REMOVAL.

Lymphoedema

This means persistent swelling of the tissues from blockage or absence of the lymph drainage vessels which carry tissue fluid (*lymph*) from the tissues back into the bloodstream. This may be caused by:

- deficiency of the lymph channels from birth, in which case it usually affects the legs
- operative removal, as in the surgical treatment of cancer
- obstruction by cancer cells
- obstruction by microscopic parasitic worms

The latter is a tropical disorder and causes elephantiasis.

Lymphoedema of the arm following surgical treatment or radiotherapy for cancer of the breast is difficult to treat. Success has been achieved, however, by tight compression with an elastic arm stocking and regular firm massage from the wrist to the armpit. It may be necessary to sleep with the arm raised in a sling above the level of the heart.

M

Mammography

Mammography is X-ray examination used in cases of suspected breast cancer and as a screening procedure for women. The value of mammography is still debated by some, but improvements in instruments and technique have increased its reliability, and most doctors now acknowledge its value. The procedure cannot be relied on to exclude cancer and does not distinguish between benign and malignant tumours. It does, however, often bring to light cases in which sampling of tissue (*biopsy*) is needed and, in this way, can lead to early diagnosis and cure of cancer.

About 40% of lumps cannot be felt, even by careful palpation, but may be detected by mammography. Of these, 20–30% contain cancer. Cysts, which are non-malignant, are easily visualized. Mammography is of little value to women under 35, but regular mammography is widely recommended for women over 50. The radiation dosage is very low and offers no significant risk.

The procedure, and position of the patient, varies with the type of machine, but is painless, although sometimes quite uncomfortable. A variety of methods is used to allow the soft tissue to be X-rayed without interference from other structures. The breasts may be laid on top of a flat surface or allowed to hang down; they may be sucked into a cavity, or may be gently squeezed between plates.

Menopause

The menopause or climacteric is the natural end of the sequence of menstrual periods and the end of the fertile years of life in a woman. The menopause occurs at an average age of about 50 but the usual range is from 48 to 54. Occurrences outside this range are quite common. A premature menopause occurs if the ovaries are removed surgically (*oophorectomy*). The menopause involves a cessation of egg production (*ovulation*) by the ovaries and of the resulting hormonal changes which alter the inner lining of the UTERUS.

The main effect of the menopause is a reduced production of the hormone oestrogen by the ovaries. Some of the symptoms and effects of the menopause are due to oestrogen deficiency, but, for some women, the awareness that they have come to the end of reproductive life and have reached a significant stage in ageing, may have as much effect as the hormone deficiency. The menopause often coincides with the departure of the last of the now grown-up children from the family home, and a mother may suffer the feeling that she is now less valued.

Most women pass easily through the menopause and are relatively unaffected. Many are relieved to be spared the risk of pregnancy or the need for contraception. About a quarter suffer in some way, mainly from hot flushes, night sweats, insomnia, headaches and general irritability. Often these symptoms are severe enough, in themselves, to justify treatment. It is by no means certain that these symptoms are due to oestrogen deficiency – this has never been proved. But the placebo effect of oestrogen treatment is strong and most women and their doctors believe it responsible for the resulting improvement.

A lack of oestrogen causes thinning of the wall of the vagina and a reduction in lubricating secretions in about a quarter of postmenopausal women. This can cause difficulty and discomfort in sexual intercourse but is easily corrected by HORMONE REPLACEMENT THERAPY (HRT), either with an oestrogen alone or with combined oestrogen and progesterone treatment. For long-term use, the latter is safer but has the disadvantage that menstrual bleeding continues. The important sign of postmenopausal bleeding – a possible indication of cancer – may be obscured.

Oestrogens are strongly protective against the major arterial and heart diseases in non-smoking women, and this protection is lost after the menopause. This is held by many to be an added justification for hormone replacement therapy. Loss of bone bulk and OSTEOPOROSIS is a natural feature of ageing, but reduced oestrogen accelerates the process in postmenopausal women. This is a strong indication for hormone replacement therapy.

Contrary to widespread belief, the menopause is not associated with a marked increase in psychiatric disturbance. Most women find, to their surprise, that conventional Western attitudes and beliefs about the menopause are exaggerated and unnecessarily alarmist. But they are part of the cultural tradition and continue to be perpetuated in spite of much evidence to the contrary.

Miscarriage

It is believed that as many as one in five pregnancies end in spontaneous miscarriage. Miscarriage may be caused by abnormal chromosomes so that a fetus, which would have grown to be an abnormal baby, is discarded. The developing fetus may implant at an unsuitable site in the uterus; the uterus may be abnormal or the neck of the uterus (*cervix*) too weak to retain the growing fetus. The mother may be producing insufficient hormones (especially progesterone) to maintain the pregnancy or there may be infection of the reproductive organs. All these can lead to miscarriage. In most cases the cause of spontaneous abortion is not identified.

The unmistakable sign of *threatened abortion* is bleeding, or a dark brown discharge, from the vagina. Often there is a slight pain, like a period pain, in the lower abdomen. Although the embryo or fetus remains alive and still attached to the wall of the uterus, the bleeding indicates that there is a threat of separation. About a quarter of these will go on to miscarriage, but most settle down, and the pregnancy continues to full term with delivery of a healthy, normal baby. In such cases, threatened abortion does not imply that there is anything wrong with the baby.

If the bleeding gets worse and the pain becomes more severe and cramping, there comes a point when it has to be recognized that miscarriage is inevitable. Inevitable abortion means that the cervix has opened and the contents of the uterus are being expelled by contractions. Blood clots and membranes, enclosing the fetus, will have passed into the vagina. Sometimes bleeding from an inevitable abortion is so severe as to call for a blood transfusion.

Often the expulsion is incomplete and a minor operation, under general anaesthesia, may be needed. This is called evacuation of retained products of conception (ERPC). The uterus is emptied by suction and the lining is carefully scraped with a sharp-edged spoon called a curette. A drug is then given to cause the uterus to contract and antibiotics may also be necessary. The patient is usually able to go home the next day.

Sometimes the fetus dies but is retained in the uterus. This is called *missed abortion*. In this case there is often a history of threatened miscarriage that has apparently settled. But later, the signs of pregnancy – morning sickness, breast enlargement and tenderness – disappear. A brownish discharge may occur. Suspicion that this has happened can be confirmed by ultrasound scanning, which will no longer show a fetal heart beat. In the end the remaining material is usually expelled spontaneously, but an ERPC is often necessary.

Most miscarriages occur in the early weeks of pregnancy. Later miscarriage is less common and may mean that there is something wrong with the uterus or that the cervix is unable to remain closed. This is described by doctors as cervical incompetence. In the latter case, the cervix opens up, with little or no pain and minimal bleeding and the baby is lost. This can usually be prevented in subsequent pregnancies by the use of a string tied around the neck of the uterus to strengthen the cervix. This is called a cervical suture.

Some women abort repeatedly and are described as 'habitual aborters'. Gynaecological investigation will reveal the cause in about 40% of cases.

Myalgic encephalitis

Encephalitis means 'inflammation of the brain' and *myalgic* means 'relating to muscle pain'. The concept of myalgic encephalitis (ME) has been the cause of much silent suffering in women. It has also deeply divided the medical profession for years and has provoked sometimes acrimonious and dismissive argument between those who believe the condition entirely imaginary and those who think it has an organic basis. The often derogatory remarks made about people with this problem and the implication that most of them are malingerers or manipulators betrays the common but somewhat outdated notion that the mind and the body are entirely separable.

There is no questioning the existence of a common and serious disorder, affecting predominantly women, that features severe fatigue and emotional disturbance. The condition is made worse by exercise, a single act of which may cause fatigue for weeks. Unfortunately, these effects have been variously associated with a great number of other symptoms and signs, and a range of names has been applied to what may or may not be the same condition. These names include the Royal Free disease, epidemic neuromyasthenia, Otago mystery disease, Icelandic disease, institutional mass hysteria, benign myalgic encephalomyelitis and the postviral fatigue syndrome.

The basic difficulty, so far as medical attitudes are concerned, stems from two points; firstly, medical awareness that complaint of persistent fatigue is often a feature of neurotic illness in which the sufferer is seeking a resolution of some major personal or social problem; and secondly, the failure of medical investigation to find a cause.

Virus infection has been widely proposed as a cause of the syndrome and a wide range of viruses including Coxsackie, herpes, polio, varicella-zoster (chickenpox and shingles) and

Epstein-Barr (glandular fever) have been cited. Unfortunately, the finding of antibodies to these or other viruses in people with ME proves nothing. The world is full of people with such antibodies who do not have ME. Moreover, psychological stress increases susceptibility to infection, so even a higher than normal prevalence of these antibodies in ME sufferers would not prove that viruses are the cause. Extensive immunological studies into people with ME have been inconclusive.

Although the condition is called an encephalitis, none of the normal neurological tests, such as electroencephalography, show that this is present. Some tests on muscle fibres have shown abnormalities in some cases but these have not been universally accepted.

It is clear that the 'fatigue' experienced by ME sufferers is not a matter of the muscles alone and is quite different from the weakness experienced in muscular disorders such as myasthenia gravis. The fatigue of ME has a strong cognitive element and is commonly associated with mild to severe depression. A comparison of the bodily effects of depression – fatigue, headache, breathlessness, chest pain, dizziness and often bowel upset – with those of ME shows a striking similarity. The prevalences of ME and of depression are also very similar. In some cases the syndrome has responded well to treatment with antidepressant drugs.

Derogatory attitudes on the part of doctors and others have not been helpful and have caused great distress to sufferers who have often been forced to turn to alternative therapists. Whether the condition is of external organic origin or otherwise is, currently, the central point at issue. But it is equally important to acknowledge that people whose lives are as severely affected as those of ME sufferers, deserve as much help as any similarly affected people, whatever the cause. Such a gross and persistent disruption of normal living indicates a major disorder of the whole person and can, in no sense, be considered to be 'all in the mind'.

Myxoedema

A term used to describe the general effects of severe underactivity of the thyroid gland. This occurs in women five times as often as in men. The skin is dry and scaly, cold, thickened and coarse. The hair is scanty, coarse and brittle. Often the eyebrows are greatly thinned or even partly absent. The lips are thickened and mauve-coloured and there is halitosis. The affected person does not complain, but is lethargic, readily fatigued, slowed in body and mind and suffers muscle aches, loss of menstruation, deafness, angina pectoris, heart failure, ANAEMIA and constipation.

All these effects can be reversed by the administration of thyroid hormones.

N

Nail disorders

Because of their position, and the constant use of the hands, fingernails are vulnerable to injury. Commonly, as a result of injury, a collection of blood (*haematoma*) forms under the nail, and this may affect nail adhesion. Detachment of the nail from its bed is called *onycholysis*. Apart from injury, onycholysis may be caused by psoriasis, fungus infection and thyroid gland overactivity. The separation usually starts at the tip and extends backwards. Air under the nail gives it a greyish-white colour. A complete, spontaneous shedding of one or more nails can occur in any severe illness as this can lead to a sudden cessation of nail growth and lack of adhesion of the plate to the bed. Toenails are also susceptible to injury, often repeated, and this may lead to a condition of very marked thickening, and claw-like curving, known as *onychogryphosis*.

Paronychia, the infection of the soft tissue around the nail, is probably the commonest of all nail disorders. It most commonly affects the toes and is popularly, but incorrectly, known as 'ingrowing toenail'. There is pain, swelling and inflammation, and sometimes pus appears at the nail edge. The condition usually results from repeated minor injury and working conditions which make proper hand care difficult. Fungus infection of the nails (*onychomycosis*) is common and causes thickening, distortion and separation. It is hard to treat but will respond to the drug griseofulvin which must be taken for at least a year. Unfortunately there may be side effects.

Small point-like depressions (pits) occur in the persistent skin disease psoriasis and in patchy baldness (*alopecia areata*). Single horizontal ridges that move along, with growth, towards the tip of the nail may indicate a previous illness. Multiple horizontal ridges suggest infection in the skin around the nail bed. Longitudinal ridges occur in alopecia areata, psoriasis and in the very itchy skin disease lichen planus. Nail thickening is common in psoriasis and fungus infection. The small white patches occurring on most people's nails have never been adequately explained.

Nipple disorders

The nipple is the central prominence of each breast, larger in women than in men. The word derives from the Anglo-Saxon *nib*, meaning 'a little beak'. In women, 15 to 20 milk ducts pass from the milk-producing lobes of the breast out through each nipple. The area surrounding the nipple is called the areola and this is a pinkish colour in those who have not been pregnant, but darker in those who have. Erection of the nipple occurs in the cold, on light touch, on sexual excitement and on the stimulus of breast feeding.

Nipples are sometimes naturally turned inwards (*inverted*) and this can cause feeding problems. Inverted nipples should be regularly pulled out. A naturally inverted nipple should be distinguished from a previously normal nipple which becomes indrawn or distorted. This may be a sign of cancer and should be reported to a doctor at once.

Cracked and sore nipples are common features of breast-feeding. Cracked nipples can allow access to infective organisms and may lead to a BREAST ABSCESS. Cracks should be allowed to heal even if breastfeeding must be stopped for a day or two and the milk expressed and given from a bottle. Sore nipples sometimes occur when the nipple is pulled from the baby's mouth instead of breaking the suction with a finger. Teething babies should be firmly stopped from biting. Sore nipples should be exposed as much as possible and allowed to dry after feeds. See also PAGET'S DISEASE OF THE NIPPLE.

O

Osteoporosis

Our bones are made mainly of a tough, elastic protein called collagen organized along efficient engineering lines to produce maximum strength with minimum weight. But bones made solely of collagen would be rubbery and useless so the entire collagen structure is reinforced and stiffened with calcium and phosphorus. If, for any reason, there is a shortage of minerals, especially calcium, the reinforcement becomes inadequate and bones will soften and may bend under the body weight. This occurs in rickets in children and osteomalacia in adults, usually because calcium is not being absorbed properly from the intestine because of a deficiency of vitamin D. In osteoporosis, however, the basic problem is not a deficiency of minerals.

Like the rest of the tissues of your body, living bones are in a state of constant physical and chemical change, losing and gaining dissolved calcium, phosphorus and the protein sub-units, the amino acids, to and from your bloodstream. The movement of these substances is controlled by various growth and sex hormones some of which reduce, and some of which increase, the amounts that are deposited in your bones. Changes in the amounts of these hormones can thus greatly affect the strength of your bones, both in mineral and in protein terms.

The sex hormones and the bones
The most important hormones in this respect are the sex hor-

mones. You probably think of the sex hormones as substances that determine gender and sexuality. This is true, but an equally important effect of the sex hormones is to make people stronger. Sex hormones, both male and female, are steroids and they are *anabolic*. The word simply means 'building up'. The sudden growth spurt at puberty and the physical changes in the body are due to sex hormones. Male sex hormones are more anabolic than female. This gives men a double advantage over women in relation to bone strength – first, because of the greater anabolic effect and second, because men go on producing their sex hormones throughout life while women stop producing them at the time of the menopause. Because of this, and because men start off with thicker bones than women, osteoporosis is essentially a woman's problem. Soon after the menopause the loss of density in women's bones tends to accelerate and in 20 years the loss can be considerable and dangerous.

Other hormones, and also hormone drugs, can affect bone strength. One of the hormones from the adrenal glands is called cortisol. This is a *catabolic* ('breaking-down') steroid and too much cortisol or other corticosteroids can be very bad for the bones and may rapidly cause osteoporosis. In the disease known as Cushing's syndrome, overproduction of cortisol by one or both adrenal glands causes osteoporosis. There is a large range of corticosteroid drugs which are identical to, or closely similar to, cortisol. These steroids also cause osteoporosis and this danger should be balanced against their importance in the management of other conditions. For this and other reasons the steroids should never be used without good reason.

In addition to the steroids, various natural body hormones control the amounts of calcium and phosphorus in the bones. Disorders of these hormone glands can lead to softening or undue hardening of the bones, as minerals are leached out or over-deposited.

Strength from use

There is another important factor that can influence the strength of your bones. Bones are thickest and strongest in early adult life, thereafter becoming gradually thinner with age as a result of progressive loss of the protein structure and of minerals. This occurs for an unexpected reason. The rate of decline in bone strength is affected to an important degree by the demands we make on them. Bones stay strong by being used and by having physical forces, such as those involved in weight-bearing, walking, running and so on, applied to them. These physical forces actually stimulate the bone-forming cells into action so that the need for greater strength is met. This is an example of the many ways in which the body reacts to external demand.

Under-use of the bones, as occurs in bed-ridden people or in astronauts living in zero gravity, leads to osteoporosis. Even a change from an active to a sedentary life as a result of arthritis or some other disabling condition, will cause osteoporosis. And, of course, the ordinary processes of ageing, with associated loss of activity and reduced hormone levels, will inevitably cause it. Women should be especially aware of the importance of keeping up the levels of activity throughout life.

The effects of osteoporosis

These are as common as they are severe. A quarter of a million thighbone neck fractures occur in the USA, and nearly 40 000 in Britain, every year. Four-fifths of these are attributable, wholly or partially, to osteoporosis. The cost of treating osteo-porosis-related medical conditions in the USA is about six bil-lion dollars a year. Unfortunately, osteoporosis causes no symptoms until some effect of the weakening in the bones occurs. The commonest effect of all is an unexpected fracture of the neck of the hip bone as a result of a quite minor stumble or fall. Thirty per cent of women over the age of 60 suffer this misfortune and the consequences are often very serious. In spite of brilliant improvements in the orthopaedic surgical management of fracture of the neck of the femur, this disaster still commonly shortens life. Twenty-five per cent of women over 60 suffer fractures of the spinal bones (*vertebrae*) as a result of osteoporosis. The extent of the problem is partly con-cealed by uncomplaining, patient women who attribute their symptoms to 'old age' and do not seek medical help.

Other effects of osteoporosis include:

- fracture of the wrist from minor stress
- persistent severe back pain
- loss of height from shrinkage of the bones of the spinal column
- sudden collapse of one of the bones of the spine with severe pain and 'dowager's hump' disfigurement
- severe and progressive curvature of the spine so that the body becomes ever more bent

Such osteoporotic spinal curvature (*kyphosis*) is disfiguring and, especially if there was a previous tendency to stooping, may sometimes become so extreme as to force the chin on to the chest and even interfere with eating. Many women become so embarrassed over their appearance that they go out as little as possible, avoid social contacts and become reclusive.

Kyphosis

An abnormal degree of backward curvature of part of the spine is called kyphosis. The term comes from the Greek *kyphos* meaning 'bowed or bent', and is used to describe a degree of backward curvature of the spine sufficient to cause deformity.

Kyphosis is due to downward loading on the spine so that the normal curves are exaggerated. This will not happen unless there is inadequate support, either from poor muscles, faulty posture or weakening of the bones. It therefore tends to affect two groups – adolescents, as a result of slouching or slumping and postmenopausal women as a result of osteoporosis. Progressive kyphosis from osteoporosis calls for energetic medical management. Neglected, the outcome may be one of serious height loss, gross deformity and sometimes major disability.

What should you do about it?

Once osteoporosis has developed it is very difficult to restore bone strength. So there are many good reasons to try to minimize the rate of loss of bone bulk. Taking regular exercise, as strenuous as is reasonable and safe, is one obvious measure you should never neglect. Taking plenty of calcium – at least 1,500 mg per day – is harmless and distinctly worthwhile. For some inexplicable reason, cigarette smoking is associated with increased osteoporosis. This is just one of the many strong reasons why smoking should be avoided. Moderation in alcohol intake is also recommended for this and other reasons.

There is now complete medical agreement that oestrogen HORMONE REPLACEMENT THERAPY (HRT) significantly reduces the risk of osteoporosis in women after the menopause. Oestrogens unquestionably retard the process of loss of bone substance, but do not lead to an increase in bone bulk. Unfortunately, they do have some disadvantages, especially in producing a slight increase in the risk of BREAST and UTERUS CANCER. In spite of this, most doctors are strongly in favour of oestrogen HRT. There is good evidence that calcium supplements in the diet also help. A recent large multinational study of the effects of oestrogens, calcium and calcitonin on women over 50 reported in the *British Medical Journal* in November, 1992, showed that all three supplements significantly reduced the risk of hip fracture.

The decision is, of course, yours, but it should be an informed decision. If you are in a category with a slight increase in the risk of breast cancer – perhaps because your mother has or had this misfortune – you may feel that the slightly increased risk should not be taken. At the same time, it is important for you to know that the mortality rate from breast cancer (as well as from other causes) is significantly lower in women on HRT than in comparable groups not taking it. If you already know, from X-ray or other scanning evidence, that you have a degree of osteoporosis and if you are a naturally small-boned person, you owe it to yourself to consider seriously what you should do to minimize the risks of future bone problems. HRT by the skin patch method is more effective and has fewer side effects than HRT by mouth. The risk of uterus cancer can be eliminated by adding proges- terone to the oestrogen.

Ovarian cancer

Cancer of the ovary is commoner in women who have never had children than in those who have. It may occur at any age but is most usual between 50 and 60. Unfortunately, ovarian cancer tends to be symptomless ('silent') until it has grown and spread, displacing and invading the UTERUS and spreading widely within the pelvis and abdomen. Diagnosis is usually made by direct viewing with a fine instrument called an endo- scope, which is passed through the wall of the abdomen.

The treatment is surgical and the uterus and both ovaries must be removed as the second ovary often also contains a tumour. Ovarian cancer is often very susceptible to anti-cancer chemotherapy. Radiotherapy is seldom useful.

Ovarian cysts

These can occur at any age, but are commonest between 35 and 55. Most of them produce no symptoms and the only sign is a gradual increase in the size of the abdomen which is often attributed to simple obesity. Ovarian cysts can become very large, however, and may press on and partially obstruct the large pelvic veins leading to varicose veins or piles (*haemor- rhoids*). They can also compress the urine tubes from the kid- neys (*ureters*) and cause kidney damage. Their sheer bulk can cause breathlessness and abdominal discomfort. Women sometimes mistake this enlargement for a pregnancy.

Cysts may be caused by slight disorders of ovulation or by

distention of the delicate outer lining of the ovary from fluid collection. Such swellings are usually harmless. Cysts caused in this way usually pass unnoticed, but occasionally they grow big enough to cause pain. Treatment is seldom required.

The commonest true ovarian cysts are called serous cysts and contain watery fluid. These occur late in the reproductive life or after the menopause and may be of almost any size up to an enormous bulk, filling and distending the abdomen. The similar pseudomucinous cysts contain a viscous mucoid fluid and may also grow very large. These cysts cause trouble mainly by their bulk, but may cause severe complications if they become twisted and their blood supply is cut off or if they rupture or become infected. Surgeons are very careful to avoid damaging the capsule when removing pseudomucinous cysts, as the contents are very irritating to the inner lining of the abdomen (*peritoneum*), and cells can be released which can set up new cysts elsewhere in the abdomen. Ovarian cysts may result from ENDOMETRIOSIS of the ovary. These contain altered blood and almost always cause pain. Surgical treatment is usually necessary.

Ovaries

These are the basic female gonads of central importance to your sexual development. Your ovaries are situated in your pelvis, one on each side of the UTERUS, just under, and inward of, the open ends of the FALLOPIAN TUBES. Your ovaries are almond-shaped and about 3 cm long, with prominent blood vessels. Each ovary contains many ovum sites known as *Graafian follicles*. Once a month, one of these, or sometimes more than one, matures, swells up a little, ruptures and

releases an ovum. This is called ovulation. Ovulation sometimes causes minor pain known as 'middle pain' or *mittelschmerz*. After ovulation, each ruptured follicle is replaced
by a yellow body known as a *corpus luteum*. In addition to producing ova, your ovaries synthesize three types of steroid hormone – oestrogens, progesterones (both of which are female
sex hormones) and androgens, which, believe it or not, are
male sex hormones. The male sex hormones are anabolic and
are quite useful in helping you to develop good muscles.
Fortunately, they are not normally able to overcome the femi-
nizing effect of the female sex hormones.

Ovum

The egg, or ovum, is the female reproductive cell (*gamete*),
produced by one or other of your ovaries about halfway
between two menstrual periods. Your ovaries usually produce
one egg per month, but may produce more than one. The egg
contains 23 of the 46 chromosomes needed to make a new
individual. The other 23 are supplied by the sperm at the
moment of fertilization. The egg is a very large cell, as cells go,
much larger than a sperm, and is about 0.1 mm in diameter.
This is by far the largest cell in your body. Like all eggs it is
large because it has to contain food (*yolk*) to keep the embryo
nourished during its earliest stages before it can establish a
supply from the mother via the placenta.

If more than one egg is produced and fertilized, a multiple
pregnancy results, but the babies are not identical because, in
each case, half the chromosomes come from different sperms,
with different genetic material. But if a fertilized ovum divides
and each of the two halves forms a new individual, these will

be identical twins, with identical chromosomes.

At birth the ovaries contain about a million immature ova. Only about four hundred of these immature ova become mature and are released. No new ova are produced after birth and all those that may be fertilized are the same age as the woman. This is why there is a slight tendency for genetic abnormalities to be commoner in babies born to older women. The ova have had longer to develop mutations.

P

Paget's disease of the nipple

It is quite common for an itchy skin rash to affect both breasts. This is often a form of eczema, calling for treatment with ointments. But if a patch of reddened skin, resembling eczema, appears on only one nipple, it is possible that, under it, is a small cancer. This may be so even if you cannot feel a lump. This is called Paget's disease of the nipple.

Such a patch should always be reported. Usually a biopsy, to exclude or confirm cancer, is required. Paget's disease does not readily spread beyond the breast tissue, but should always be removed. Undue delay is dangerous. There is also a Paget's disease of bone, but this is quite a different condition.

Pelvic examination

This is often called 'vaginal examination', but the gynaecologist is not so much concerned with the vagina as with what may be felt in the pelvis by way of the vagina. This examination involves both hands, the second being used to feel through the front wall of your abdomen. Pelvic examination is often quite uncomfortable, and if there are any inflamed parts within your pelvis, pressure on them will cause pain. The doctor wants to know about this, so being brave is not particularly helpful. The important thing, however, is to try to relax everything as much as you can. This will make it easier for you and the doctor.

Direct visual examination of the interior of the pelvis is

called laparoscopy. This is done using fibreoptic illumination and viewing channels contained in a narrow viewing tube (*endoscope*), which can be passed through a small cut in the wall of your abdomen. Laparoscopy can be used by any specialist concerned with disease of the abdominal organs, but has been especially adopted by gynaecologists for the investigation of disorders of the female reproductive organs in the pelvis. Conditions, such as ectopic pregnancy, and sterility from possible obstruction of the fallopian tubes, which are difficult to diagnose with certainty in any other way short of an exploratory abdominal operation, can be diagnosed in this way. Laparoscopy also allows a range of operations to be performed and is widely used as a means of deliberately closing off the fallopian tubes to achieve sterilization. Laparoscopy can be valuable in the diagnosis of doubtful cases of appendicitis, or diseases of the gall bladder or liver.

Laparoscopy is usually done under general anaesthesia. Harmless carbon dioxide gas is passed in through a small needle to inflate the abdominal cavity and move the intestines out of the way. The endoscope can then be safely inserted through a small incision. Various instruments, including laser channels, can be passed through the laparoscope, for diverse purposes. In particular, tissues can be vaporized and cut, without bleeding; local disease, such as patches of ENDOMETRIOSIS, destroyed; and biopsies can be taken from any organ, including the liver. Eggs (*ova*) can be taken from the ovaries for *in vitro fertilization* (see INFERTILITY). The pressure of the gas in the abdomen may cause some discomfort for a day or two, until it absorbs. There may also be referred pain from irritation of the diaphragm. This is felt in the tip of the shoulder.

In videolaseroscopy or videoendoscopy, a video camera is attached to the laparoscope so that the interior of the abdomen can be viewed on a TV monitor and the procedure carried out while watching the screen. This is convenient for the surgeon who, in the past, has had to spend long periods bending over the patient's abdomen looking through a single small eyepiece. Zoom magnification of small areas is possible and videotape recordings can be made.

Pelvis

The pelvis is the bony girdle formed by the two hip bones on either side and the triangular curved sacrum, behind. The hip bones are held together in front by a midline joint called the pubic symphysis. Behind, each hip bone is attached to the sacrum at one of the two sacroiliac joints. Each hip bone contains a deep, spherical cup, called the acetabulum, into which the head of the thigh bone (*femur*) fits.

The sacroiliac joints are the semi-rigid ligamentous junctions, at the back, holding the two outer bones of the pelvis to the side surfaces of the sacrum. The coccyx, or tail bone, consists of four small vertebrae fused together and joined to the curved sacrum. Normally very little movement occurs at the sacroiliac joints, but late in pregnancy the strong ligaments holding the joints together become more lax, so as to allow easier childbirth. The width of your hips depends on the width of your pelvis and on the angle with which the heads of your two thigh bones articulate with it.

Experts can easily distinguish a female pelvis from a male, by its proportions. The female pelvis is relatively wider and shallower than the male and the lower opening (the outlet) is better shaped to allow a baby's head to pass. The lower part of the sacrum is also more flexible in the female.

Period problems

Since menstruation is the result of hormonal influences on a structure which is, itself, liable to a variety of diseases, the range of menstrual disorders is considerable.

Premenstrual tension (PMT)

This is a state of heightened mental tension with various physical symptoms that affects some women between the time of ovulation and the start of the next period. The symptoms improve as soon as the period has started and usually pass altogether until about ten days before the next period. It mainly affects women over 30. Symptoms of PMT include:

- a general feeling of illness (*malaise*)
- irritability or anger
- depression
- loss of concentration
- loss of energy
- insomnia or over-sleeping
- backache
- discomfort in the pelvis
- a sense of bloating
- headache
- soreness of the breasts
- weight gain of up to 1 kg

The weight gain is due to fluid and salt retention. Medical opinion is divided on the reality or significance of PMT but many women will testify that they suffer badly at this time. PMT has been accepted as a legal defence on the grounds of diminished responsibility, but this fact is of no medical significance. Some doctors think that PMT is due to a relative over-production of oestrogen, compared with progesterone, in the second half of the cycle.

Maybe you can persuade your doctor to prescribe a drug to encourage urination (a *diuretic* such as chlorothiazide) so as to get rid of the surplus water. This can give you a lot of relief. Progesterone by injection or by mouth will also relieve premenstrual tension in many cases. A mild tranquillizer may be necessary.

Painful menstruation

This is called dysmenorrhoea and is very common, having been experienced by almost all women from time to time. Just before, or at the beginning of the period, there is cramping, rhythmical pain in the lower abdomen and back, lasting usually for a few hours, but sometimes for a day, or even throughout the period. The pain is associated with strong contractions of the UTERUS and with opening (*dilatation*) of the neck of the uterus (*cervix*). There may also be nausea, vomiting, diarrhoea, and cramping, colicky pain in the bowels. Some women have faintness and dizziness. In about 10% it is severe enough to cause temporary disability.

Dysmenorrhoea is almost always cured by having a baby, but less drastic remedies can also be effective. Drugs of the antiprostaglandin type (Brufen, Panadol and Aspirin) are useful, and in severe cases, menstruation can be stopped altogether by means of oral contraceptives, taken continuously. This should be done only under medical supervision.

The condition may also result as a secondary effect of pelvic infection and other local disease, such as uterine fibroids or ENDOMETRIOSIS and, in these cases, antibiotics for infection or surgery may be necessary to effect a cure.

Absence of periods

Amenorrhoea is the absence of menstruation and this may be primary (in girls of menstrual age who have not started to menstruate) or secondary, in those who have already had periods. Primary amenorrhoea may be due to hormonal causes, stress, or an imperforate hymen which completely closes off the vaginal outlet. The commonest cause of secondary amenorrhoea is, of course, pregnancy, but after that amenorrhoea is probably most often caused by ANOREXIA NERVOSA or by severe nutritional inadequacy. Amenorrhoea also occurs in athletes engaged in sustained, very vigorous training. Oligomenorrhea means infrequent or scanty periods.

Too much bleeding (menorrhagia)

Menorrhagia means excessive bleeding during periods occurring at normal intervals. Polymenorrhea means having periods more often than every three weeks. Metrorrhagia is bleeding between periods.

Heavy periods lasting for seven or eight days with frequent passage of clots are normal for some women and may continue throughout the menstrual life. But if your normal period is three to four days of light bleeding and bleeding such as this were to occur, this would represent menorrhagia. In any case, a period requiring a change of tampon or pad every hour, for more than a few hours, indicates an abnormality likely to require medical attention.

Menorrhagia is most commonly due to an excessive build-up of the endometrium – the inner lining of the UTERUS – and this is controlled by oestrogen. Progesterone, which comes from the follicle in the ovary after the ovum is released, controls the bleeding. At the beginning and the end of the menstrual life, periods often occur without ovulation, so in the absence of progesterone, the periods may be very heavy. Progesterone may be used to control this type of menorrhagia.

Another cause of heavy vaginal bleeding is spontaneous abortion and this often occurs without pregnancy being suspected. Up to 10% of pregnancies end in this way, and the retained products may cause heavy bleeding. In this case, the bleeding can be stopped by a DILATATION AND CURETTAGE (D and C).

Fibroid tumours and polyps may cause excessive bleeding, as may cancer of the endometrium of the uterus, but the latter is likely to cause irregular bleeding, rather than menorrhagia.

Irregularity

A misleading term used to describe the effect of a variety of influences, including the occasional missed periods that occur normally at the beginning of the menstrual life and at the time of the MENOPAUSE. A common cause of apparent irregularity is pregnancy followed by MISCARRIAGE at a very early stage. Often, pregnancy may be unsuspected.

Periods missed as a result of anorexia, excessive dieting, or strenuous athletics may also cause an apparent irregularity. Another common cause is midcycle bleeding, when, at the time of ovulation, oestrogen levels may briefly drop sufficiently to allow the uterus lining to break down.

The appearance of menstrual irregularity may result from abnormal bleeding from other causes. When there is inflammation of the vagina or cervix, bleeding may occur after intercourse. Bleeding may result from trauma to polyps or tumours. It may also be due to ENDOMETRIOSIS, to cancer of the endometrium or to the presence of an IUD (*intrauterine contraceptive device*).

Pessary

A pessary is a small medicated vaginal plug or suppository, usually containing a drug, an antiseptic or a spermicide. The active substance is dissolved in a waxy vehicle, such as coconut butter, that melts at body temperature. This is a convenient and effective way of applying medication to the vagina.

The term is also used to describe one of various devices, often ring-shaped, inserted in the vagina to correct downward displacement (*prolapse*) or retroversion of the uterus. Another type, the diaphragm pessary, is used as a barrier method of contraception.

Phobias

These are intense, irrational fears which cannot be ignored or overcome even when the sufferer is fully aware, as is usually the case, that there is no reason for the fear. Phobias take many forms and include fear of humiliation or embarrassment (social phobias), fear of high places (*acrophobia*), fear of open places (*agoraphobia*), fear of spiders (*arachnophobia*), fear of enclosed places (*claustrophobia*), fear of cats (*gatophobia*), fear of water (*hydrophobia*), fear of dead bodies (*necrophobia*), fear of darkness (*nyctophobia*), fear of crowds (*ochlophobia*) and fear of animals (*zoophobia*).

Phobias may relate to almost any situation, idea or object and most people have at least one mild phobia. Severe phobias are, however, very disabling and can seriously disrupt normal living. Most people have a reasonable fear of cancer, but cancer phobia has nothing to do with reason. It is a distressing personality disorder of the *phobic* type, with the attention of the affected person directed towards cancer.

Cancer phobia, unfortunately, does not prompt the sufferer to rational courses such as regular breast screening, BREAST SELF-EXAMINATION, CERVICAL SMEAR TESTS (*Pap smears*), avoidance of risk factors such as smoking, and so on. Instead, it gives rise to compulsively performed rituals, especially repeated handwashing, changing of clothes that have been touched by others, avoidance of air breathed by others, and even avoidance of any contact with other people. Symptoms, however minor, are interpreted as signs of cancer and panic attacks may occur. As with any other phobic disorder, cancer phobia cannot be treated by appeals to the reason.

The cause of phobias remains obscure but it seems likely that they are simple, forgotten conditioned reflexes which are kept active (*reinforced*) by the repeated drive to avoid the unpleasant experience. This view is supported by the success of behaviour therapy in removing phobias. The physiological responses to phobias – fast pulse, sweating, high blood pressure, and so on, can be controlled by the use of beta-blocking drugs.

Pica

This is a persistent tendency to eat non-nutritional substances such as earth, ice, match-heads, coal, chalk or wood. Pica is common in children under 18 months of age and, in these, is not considered abnormal. Pica in pregnancy has been known throughout the ages and the bizarre catalogue of substances eaten include mothballs, soap, insects, clay, baking soda and excrement. Pica is a feature of nutritional deficiency and iron-deficiency anaemia and sometimes succeeds in providing a needed supply of minerals. It will often stop if anaemia is effectively treated.

In most cases, pica does little harm, but there have been many medical reports of obstruction or perforation of the bowel, lead poisoning, parasite infestation and other misfortunes from this cause. No satisfactory explanation of many types of pica has been produced.

Prolapse

The displacement, often downwards, of the whole or part of an organ, from its normal position. Prolapse occurs because of weakness or laxity of some supporting structures, such as muscles or tendons. The commonest examples of prolapse are of the rectum and UTERUS, but the bladder may prolapse into the vagina; a haemorrhoid may prolapse through the anus; or the umbilical cord may prolapse from the uterus during or before birth.

R

Rhesus factor disease

After the A, B, AB and O blood groups, the rhesus factor is the most important. The gene that makes a person rhesus positive is called D. This is present in 85% of the population. The gene is dominant, so a person is rhesus positive even if only one of the gene pair is D. All the offspring of a rhesus positive father with two D genes (*homozygous*) will be rhesus positive. If the father has only one D gene (*heterozygous*) and the mother is rhesus negative, each pregnancy will have a 50% chance of producing a rhesus positive baby.

When a rhesus positive father produces a rhesus positive baby in a rhesus negative mother, the baby's red blood cells will act as antigens capable of causing the mother to produce antibodies against them. These antigens do not normally reach the mother's blood until labour so they are unlikely to cause serious harm in the first pregnancy. But in subsequent pregnancies, the levels of these antibodies in the mother's blood rise rapidly and soon reach a point at which they are able to destroy the red cells of the fetus.

The severity of the effects on the baby vary considerably. In the most severe cases, the fetus dies in the UTERUS, usually after the 28th week. If born alive, the child may be deeply jaundiced with an enlarged liver and spleen and a low haemoglobin level in the red blood cells (*anaemia*). Excess free haemoglobin in the blood leads to excess bile pigment (*bilirubin*) production and this has a much more serious effect than merely to stain the skin and cause jaundice. Bilirubin is very toxic to the brain, which becomes bile-stained (*kernicterus*) and leads to paralysis, spasticity, mental retardation and defects of sight and hearing.

A badly affected baby can have an exchange transfusion, via the umbilical cord, as soon as it is born, or even while still in the uterus. This corrects the anaemia and gets rid of the bilirubin. Exposure to intense blue light soon after birth assists in converting the bilirubin in the skin to a form which is harmless to the brain.

Rhesus negative women can be prevented from developing antibodies by being given an injection of anti D gamma globulin within 60 hours of the birth of a rhesus positive baby. In order to protect future babies, this is done in all such cases. Gamma globulin is also given when there has been a MISCARRIAGE or if there is any other reason to believe that rhesus positive fetal blood may have gained access to the woman's circulation, as in obstetrical procedures like turning the baby (*external version*). The injection is given if an AMNIOCENTESIS shows bloodstained amniotic fluid, and is routine after an amniocentesis in a rhesus negative woman.

S

Sexual problems

Sexual activity encompasses physical, psychological, social and aesthetic elements. Anything as complex as this is liable to a range of disorders. These disorders may be apparent only to one member of a partnership or to both, and may be attributed by either to the other or to the unsatisfactory nature of the relationship. The latter is one of the most common causes of trouble. It is unreasonable to expect a good sexual rapport between people who dislike one another or who are concerned primarily with their own personal satisfaction rather than with that of the other. Fear of pregnancy, sexual ignorance, and guilt induced by misinformation and religious instruction are other major causes of sexual problems.

The proportion of sexual problems attributable to organic or structural disorder is small: the great majority are of psychological or inter-relational origin. They include:

- impotence
- ejaculatory disorders, especially premature ejaculation
- lack of orgasm in females
- inability to relax the muscles of the genitalia (*vaginismus*)
- various forms of sexual deviation

Organic disease such as neurologically- or diabetically-induced impotence, penile distortion (*Peyronie's disease*) in males, or vaginal dryness or shrinkage of the vagina in the elderly woman, can cause serious sexual difficulties.

Painful sexual intercourse

The medical term for this is dyspareunia, a word that derives
from the Greek *dyspareunos* meaning 'ill-mated'. This is a little
hard on the woman who is usually suffering from a gynaecological disorder such as an imperforate or thick, persistent
hymen, vulvitis, vaginitis, bartholinitis, urethritis, episiotomy
scars, vaginal dryness, senile or post-radiational atrophy of
the vagina, or, rarely, a congenital central vaginal partition
(*septate*, or double, vagina).

Dyspareunia is often caused by vaginal spasm (*vaginismus*)
which may be of such degree that even a finger can barely be
admitted. This condition is of psychological origin and is usually caused by fear of sex or by disinclination for sexual intercourse with a particular partner. Vaginismus is a major reflex
spasm, which may involve not only all the muscles of the
pelvis, but also the muscles which press the thighs together.
Treatment is often difficult and may, in some cases, be inappropriate. Psychotherapy, skilled counselling and patient
explanation, relaxation training, genital self-familiarization,
and the use, by the affected woman, of progressively larger
smooth, rounded dilators, may be needed. What is *not* needed
is male assertiveness and force. This causes pain, and exacer-
bates the basic causal factors.

Non-consummation

This means failure to achieve penetration of the vagina with
the penis. This is commoner than is generally supposed and is
believed to be the fate of about one marriage in 100.

Non-consummation occasionally results from ignorance on
the part of both partners, remarkable in these outspoken days,

as to what should go where. More commonly, it results from physical or psychological problems. The man may suffer impotence, of whatever sort, failure to maintain the erection, premature ejaculation or penile abnormality. The woman may have an anatomical abnormality of the vagina or a thick, rigid hymen, or, most commonly, the condition of vaginismus (see above).

Skin cancer

Many skin cancers are related to long-term exposure to sunlight. This is especially so in the cases of basal cell carcinoma (*rodent ulcer*), squamous cell carcinoma, which may develop in an area of actinic keratosis, and malignant melanoma in white people. These three conditions occur in that order of frequency, but, fortunately, the commonest, the basal cell carcinoma, is the least malignant, and the rarest, the melanoma, the most serious. Bowen's disease, which is a very slow-growing cancer within the epidermis, may also be related to sunlight exposure.

About one cancer in a hundred is a malignant melanoma. Skin melanomas are very rare in childhood and are commonest in the middle-aged and the elderly. About half of them arise from pre-existing moles. Nearly everyone has pigmented moles but only one in a million becomes malignant. Hairy moles hardly ever turn into malignant melanomas.

Malignant change in a mole can be detected by various signs. These include:

- change in shape, especially increasing irregularity of outline
- change in size

- increased protuberance beyond the surface
- change in colour, especially sudden darkening and the development of coloured irregularities appearing as different shades of brown, grey, pink, red and bluish
- itching or pain
- softening
- crumbling
- the development of new 'satellite' moles around the original one

The most dangerous melanomas are those that become nodular. This is because these tend to penetrate deeply.

Melanomas are commonest on areas exposed to the sun, but may occur anywhere on the skin. Once your suspicion has been aroused, you should never delay reporting the condition for an expert opinion. Melanomas are removed with a wide area of normal-seeming tissue around them and skin grafting may be necessary to cover the defect.

Skin disorders

The skin is at least as susceptible to disease as any other organ and the range of disorders is wide. The discipline dealing with skin disorders is called dermatology. The term *dermatitis* does not, as is commonly thought, refer to a particular condition. It simply means 'inflammation of the skin' and covers all skin disorders in which the skin is inflamed.

Many cases of dermatitis are caused by:

- infection by almost any kind of organism – viruses, bacteria, fungi and protozoa
- allergy to a wide range of contact materials

- physical or chemical injury
- damage by heat, intense ultraviolet light, or by other forms of radiation

The term *eczema* is roughly synonymous with *dermatitis*. Urticaria (*hives*) is the common skin reaction to allergy, whether from contact or ingestion.

Bacterial infection by staphylococci causes pustules, boils and carbuncles, and infection by streptococci causes spreading skin inflammation (*cellulitis*). Both staphylococci and streptococci can cause impetigo. Virus infections of the skin include cold sores and venereal herpes from herpes simplex viruses and most forms of warts. In shingles – herpes zoster – the virus is usually acquired early in life, when it causes chickenpox. Fungus infection, or epidermophytosis, causes the various forms of tinea – athlete's foot (*tinea pedis*), crutch infection (*tinea cruris*), body infection (*tinea corporis*) and ringworm of the scalp (*kerion*). Fungus also commonly infects the nails.

Infestation with various mite and insect parasites, such as the scabies mite, *Sarcoptes scabei*, fleas, bed bugs and lice, cause damage to the skin and this is often compounded by damage and secondary infection from scratching.

Birth-marks, or naevi, may take several different forms, including the port-wine stain caused by enlargement of capillaries (very small blood vessels) and pigmented moles. See also SKIN CANCER.

Common acne with the formation of blackheads (*comedones*) is related to the local action, on the sebaceous glands of the skin, of androgens (male sex hormones). A combined antiandrogen/oestrogen pill is often valuable in the management. Although it is not an infection, acne can be treated effectively a tetracycline antibiotic. Regular washing with soap and water and the use of a chlorhexidine scrub, such as Hibiscrub, are also helpful. The most effective treatment of all is the drug isotretinoin, but this can cause severe fetal abnormalities and young women who are proposing to use it must have a negative pregnancy test and must use an oral contraceptive for a month before the course, during it, and for three months afterwards.

A wen (*sebaceous cyst*) is an accumulation of sebaceous material within the skin, following the blockage of a pore.

A scar is an area of fibrous tissue which has replaced normal skin during the healing of a deep injury. Such fibrous tissue contracts on maturation, causing depression of the surface.

Psoriasis is a very common and persistent skin disease with a complex cause. It features well-demarcated, oval, reddish patches with scaly surfaces and may vary markedly in severity at different times.

Xanthelasma features yellowish plaques in the skin due to deposition of cholesterol. These commonly occur in the eyelids and do not necessarily imply raised blood cholesterol levels.

Excessive BLUSHING may herald the condition of rosacea, in which the small blood vessels of the face have an abnormal tendency to dilate.

Purpura is a condition of leaky blood vessels so that blood is released into the tissues. In the skin this may cause tiny pinpoints or dots (*petechiae*) or larger bruises.

Vitiligo is characterized by pure white patches in the skin, particularly noticeable in non-white or suntanned people. It is believed to be caused by an autoimmune destruction of the pigment cells.

Prickly heat is caused by high temperatures and humidity which lead to blockage of the ducts of sweat glands, so that small papules form.

A common cause of acceleration of skin degeneration is undue exposure to ultraviolet light. Sunbathing is a major cause of collagen damage with loss of skin elasticity and excessive wrinkling. Keratosis is also commonly caused by solar radiation and may lead to skin cancer. Other forms of radiation, such as X-rays, may cause severe injury to the skin and may eventually lead to cancer.

Striae

Striae are broad lines, called stretch marks, on the skin of the abdomen, thighs and breasts. They are red at first and slightly raised, but later become purplish and flattened. About three quarters of pregnant women develop striae and, unfortunately, because they involve damage to the elastic collagen in the skin, striae are permanent. They do, however, become very much less obvious with the passage of time, and eventually are often barely visible.

T

Tamoxifen

Tamoxifen is a remarkable drug with a very persistent effect that prevents oestrogens from acting normally in the body. It has been in use since 1971 to help to treat breast cancer in over three million women. The drug delays relapse and prolongs survival in 20–30% of affected women. Many thousands of these women have survived for more than 10 years.

There is much current interest in whether the drug is effective in preventing high-risk women from developing breast cancer. Trials of the drug in the USA, Italy, Australia and Britain, suggest that it may be a valuable preventive. In women who have had one primary breast cancer the drug appears to reduce the incidence of a second cancer by about 40%. The anti-oestrogen effects appear, on the whole, to be beneficial rather than otherwise. Older women taking the drug enjoy a 60% reduction in death from heart attacks and are significantly protected against postmenopausal osteoporosis. Pre-menopausal women have not been found to suffer such effects as an early menopause, loss of sexual interest or vaginal dryness. Some side effects are inevitable and some women taking the drug experience hot flushes, nausea, fluid retention, irregularity of menstruation and vaginal discharge. None of these effects should weigh heavily in the light of the advantages. Tamoxifen stimulates egg release (*ovulation*) and is often used in the treatment of infertility.

In Spring 1992 the American National Cancer Institute recruited 16,000 healthy women, deemed to be at high risk of breast cancer, into a tamoxifen trial. Half of these women are acting as controls and are taking an inactive placebo; half are taking the active drug. None of them know whether what they are taking is the drug or the dummy. The trial is expected to last for five years. Some doctors have criticized trials of this kind, pointing out that tamoxifen is not as harmless as many suggest. The fact that large multinational trials are being mounted by people who are well aware of these risks does, however, suggest that the majority consider the risks worth taking.

Thrush

Infection of warm, moist areas of the body with the common fungus of the genus *Candida*. Most cases are caused by the species *Candida albicans* which causes thrush of the mouth or vagina and occasionally elsewhere on the skin. Candida thrives best in darkness when the temperatures are right and especially when there is a good supply of carbohydrate for its nutrition. Candidiasis of the female vulva is thus particularly common if there is diabetes, in which there is sugar in the urine. So a urine test is mandatory in all such cases.

Fungus infections tend to be kept in check by the presence of normal body bacteria (*commensal organisms*) and if these are too energetically attacked by antibiotics, fungi may get the upper hand and start to spread.

Vaginal thrush is easily recognized. There is persistent itching or soreness and sometimes a burning pain on contact between urine and affected areas. Inspection shows characteristic white patches, rather like soft cheese, with raw-looking inflamed areas in between. There may be a white, cheesy vaginal discharge. Vulval candidiasis is easily transmitted to a sexual partner, and men, especially if uncircumcized, often develop white patches and inflammation on the glans of the penis. This is called balanitis and there is constant discomfort, varying from mild to severe.

Apart from involvement of these areas, candidiasis is uncommon in otherwise healthy people. It flourishes, however, in people whose immune systems are in any way defective. In AIDS, candidiasis spreads widely both outside and inside the body, extending from the mouth and the anal region well into both ends of the intestinal tract. Even more seriously, it often spreads into the respiratory passages and the lungs.

Candidiasis is treated with one of a range of antifungal drugs in the form of ointments, creams, meltable bullets for insertion in the vagina (*pessaries*) or drugs taken by mouth. Anti-thrush drugs include Canesten (clotrimazole), Daktarin (miconazole), Nystan (nystatin) and Diflucan (fluconazole). Thrush can be cured with a single dose of the latter drug. Treating only one of a pair of sexual partners, however, is a waste of time. This has to be a joint effort.

Thyroid gland disorders

Women are far more often troubled by thyroid gland disorders than men. This goes for both overaction and underaction of the gland. The thyroid hormones, thyroxine and tri-iodo-thyronine, act on all the cells in the body which are consuming energy, to speed up the processes of fuel consumption.

Normally, the amount of thyroid hormone in the blood is carefully controlled so that these metabolic processes occur at a correct rate. In thyroid overaction (*thyrotoxicosis*, or *hyperthyroidism*) there is excessive production of thyroid hormones, so that all these cellular processes are accelerated. In most cases the gland is either generally enlarged or contains many nodules of overactive thyroid tissue. The causes of thyrotoxicosis have not been fully explained.

Thyrotoxicosis causes:

- a marked speeding up of many of the bodily processes
- loss of weight in spite of good appetite and large intake
- rapid heart rate
- irregular pulse
- palpitation
- tremor
- sweating
- dislike of hot weather
- frequent bowel actions
- anxiety and inability to relax

A common feature is a staring appearance of the eyes, caused by a marked retraction of the upper lids. Sometimes, the eyes may protrude markedly (EXOPHTHALMOS) as a result of swelling of the tissues behind them, but this may occur long after the acute illness has subsided. Thyroid function tests show abnormal levels of the thyroid hormones in the blood.

Thyrotoxicosis is treated with drugs, such as carbimazole, methimazole and thiouracil, which cut down the activity of the gland, and sometimes by surgical removal of part of the gland (*partial thyroidectomy*). Gland activity can also be reduced by the use of a radioactive isotope of iodine. While treatment is having effect, many of the symptoms can be relieved by the use of beta-blocker drugs.

Underaction of the thyroid gland in the adult, usually the result of autoimmune diseases such as HASHIMOTO'S THYROID-ITIS, is known as hypothyroidism. This features:

- an overall slowing of the physical and mental processes
- sensitivity to cold
- obesity
- absence of sweating with scaly dry skin
- loss of hair
- puffiness of the face
- premature ageing
- coronary artery disease
- an eventual descent, unless treatment is given, into immobility and coma

Thyroid hormone, given early enough, will restore normality.

Enlargement of the thyroid gland, from any cause, is called GOITRE. Some small degree of goitre often occurs, as a normal event, around puberty or during pregnancy, but this usually settles without treatment.

Thyroid cancer is comparatively rare and presents as a single firm lump in the neck around the Adam's apple (*larynx*). If more than one lump is felt, the condition is unlikely to be cancer, but all lumps in this area must be properly investigated. Cancers grow gradually to form an increasing, irregular mass which is adherent to the adjacent structures and which spreads quickly to the lymph nodes in the neck. The nerves supplying the muscles of the vocal cords in the larynx may be involved, causing severe hoarseness or loss of the voice. Spread of the cancer to the gullet (*oesophagus*) may cause diffi-culty in swallowing.

Thyroid cancer is treated by surgical removal, by giving thyroid hormone, which restricts tumour growth, or by the use of radioactive iodine, which concentrates in the thyroid gland and in any secondary deposits of thyroid cancer else-where in the body.

Toxic shock syndrome

This is an acute, dangerous, but fortunately rare, condition caused by the absorption into the bloodstream of toxins (*tox-aemia*) from bacteria of the *Staphylococcus aureus* species. An epidemic of the toxic shock syndrome occurred among young menstruating women in the early 1980s and the condition was found to be associated with high-absorbency vaginal tampons and a rise in the staphylococci in the vagina.

The organism *S. aureus* produces three different kinds of toxins and these produce three different syndromes – food poisoning, the *scalded skin syndrome* in newborn babies and small children, and the toxic shock syndrome. Ninety per cent of cases of the toxic shock syndrome occur in menstruating women. The others occur in people with severe staphylococ-cal infections of the bone or the heart valves, or following operations.

There is a fever of 40 °C or above, an acute drop in blood pressure, a rash which becomes scaly, vomiting, diarrhoea, muscle pain, inflammation of the vagina, liver damage and sometimes disorientation and confusion. The mortality is about 2%.

TOXIC SHOCK SYNDROME

Because the trouble is caused by the toxins which have already been released from the organisms, killing the staphylococci with antibiotics has little effect on the course of the illness. It does, however, reduce the likelihood of recurrence and such treatment is always given. The use of high absorbency tampons must be avoided and all tampons should be changed frequently. It is especially important to remove the last tampon at the end of a period.

U

Urinary problems

The commonest bladder disorder is CYSTITIS – an infection more frequent in women than in men because of readier access of organisms by way of the much shorter urethra – the tube that carries urine from the bladder to the exterior.

Involuntary urination (INCONTINENCE) is another common bladder problem. It takes various forms, the most frequent in adults being *stress incontinence* in which a small quantity of urine is passed whenever the pressure within the abdomen is suddenly increased, as in coughing or laughing.

Excessive urination

Production of excessive quantities of urine, or *polyuria*, may simply be due to the excessive intake of fluid, but it is commonly a sign of diseases such as diabetes mellitus, diabetes insipidus or certain diseases of the kidney, known as *salt-losing* states. Excessive urine output also occurs when oedema from any cause is treated with diuretic drugs to get rid of the excess fluid accumulated in the tissues of the body.

Excessive urination should be distinguished from over-frequent passage of small quantities of urine, as may occur in bladder infections (cystitis).

Painful urination

Discomfort or pain on urination, usually described as 'burning' or 'scalding', is called *dysuria*. This is often associated with difficulty in starting or a sense of incomplete emptying with a desire to continue. Painful urination is most commonly caused by bladder infection (*cystitis*), but may be due to urethritis, candidiasis of the vulva, bladder polyps, bladder cancer, stone in the bladder, or the passage of blood clots or small urinary stones. Even highly concentrated urine, as may occur in fever or excessive fluid loss in sweat, may cause discomfort.

Urine retention

Inability to urinate is rare in women. Retention of urine may, however, be due to a nerve disorder. This may be a transient effect on bladder control, induced by a surgical operation, a general or spinal anaesthetic, or the use of drugs which act on the bladder or the urinary sphincters; or it may arise from actual organic disease of the spinal cord or of the nerves supplying the bladder.

Urinary retention may also be due to psychological causes or may result from narrowing of the urethra from infection or pressure from uterine fibroids, or obstruction from cancer.

Uterus

The womb or uterus is a hollow, pear-shaped organ about 8 cm long before childbirth and larger after. It has a thick, muscular wall and lies between the bladder and the rectum supported by ligaments. The lower part, the cervix, protrudes into the vagina.

The inner lining, the endometrium, is soft and velvety and contains many blood vessels and mucous glands. This lining changes considerably in the course of the menstrual cycle and much of it is cast off during menstruation. The two FALLOPIAN TUBES emerge at the upper, front end of the uterus, on either side.

Congenital abnormalities of the uterus affect about one woman in a hundred. Most of these are minor and unimportant, but sometimes the uterus is absent, doubled, or divided into two separate halves by a partition. Infections of the lining of the uterus may follow trauma, as in attempts at illegal abortion, or childbirth. Cervicitis may be caused by gonorrhoea, syphilis or a chlamydial or herpes infection. Cervical erosion is a misnomer, is common and is usually unimportant.

Functional disorders of the lining of the uterus are mostly menstrual disorders of endocrine origin. Overgrowth and atrophy are common as is the growth of areas of uterine lining (*endometrium*) elsewhere in the abdomen (ENDOMETRIOSIS). See also HYSTERECTOMY, UTERUS DISPLACEMENT (PROLAPSE), UTERUS CANCER, UTERUS FIBROIDS, UTERUS RETROVERSION.

Uterus cancer

Cancer of the lining of the UTERUS (*endometrium*) occurs most often in women between the ages of 50 and 70, and is commoner in those who have not had children. It affects mostly those who have high blood levels of oestrogen. It is much less common than cancer of the neck of the uterus (*cervix*). The first sign is usually irregular bleeding from the vagina or a blood-stained discharge. A DILATATION AND CURETTAGE (D and C) is necessary for diagnosis, and if the diagnosis has been made reasonably early and HYSTERECTOMY is performed, the outlook is usually excellent.

Cancer of the cervix is the second most common cancer in women, after BREAST CANCER. After falling steadily for many years, the incidence and mortality have now started to rise steeply, in young women in Britain. It is a common cause of death in women and is becoming commoner. Half of all cancers of the female reproductive system are in the cervix.

The disease is most likely to occur in women with a history of sexually transmitted disease, especially genital warts, women who have had many sexual partners, or whose sexual partner has genital warts, women who smoke heavily, who became pregnant at an early age and who have had three or more pregnancies. It is commonly symptomless until advanced and may cause no symptoms at all before reaching an incurable stage. Sometimes there is bleeding between periods or following sexual intercourse, but there are no dramatic early signs. Pain and general upset are rare until a late stage.

For these reasons, cancer of the cervix has to be looked for. Cervical smear screening for the pre-cancerous stage, should, ideally, be done on all women. Practical considerations dictate some restrictions, but ideally, all women should have the test at least every five years, or more often if abnormalities are found or if they are especially at risk.

Fully established cancer is difficult to treat successfully and there is no firm agreement on whether surgery or radiotherapy is best. Early cancer is commonly treated by surgery. Radiotherapy can be used at any stage. The curability depends on the extent of spread at the time of diagnosis. Early cancer, confined to the cervix, offers an excellent prognosis, with a cure rate of over 85%. But if there has been spread to the vagina and surrounding tissues, the cure rate drops to about 50%. Extensive spread to the organs of the pelvis and remote spread to other parts of the body, has a very poor outlook. In only about 10% of such cases is the patient still alive five years later.

Uterus displacement (prolapse)

The UTERUS is held in position by supporting ligaments attached to the pelvis. These can be stretched and permanently lengthened during pregnancy, especially by repeated pregnancies, and this may allow the uterus to telescope down into the vagina (*first degree prolapse*) or even to protrude beyond the vaginal opening (*second degree*). In a third degree prolapse the whole UTERUS remains outside and the surface becomes dried, whitened and thickened.

Prolapse of the uterus is often accompanied by an unpleasant feeling of lack of support or of 'something coming down'. In descending, the uterus turns the vagina outside-in and displaces the back wall of the bladder, which is immediately in front of the vaginal wall. This leads to urinary problems including INCONTINENCE and infection.

Prolapse of the uterus is treated by surgical strengthening of the supporting structures or, in severe cases, by removal of the uterus (HYSTERECTOMY). Sometimes a ring pessary can be used to keep the UTERUS in position.

Uterus fibroids

Tumours of the body of the UTERUS are common and most of them are benign i.e., not cancers. The commonest tumours are fibroids (*leiomyomas*), which affect 10% of women of reproductive age. They are benign growths of smooth muscle and fibrous tissue, of widely varying size, which may be symptomless or may cause abnormal bleeding. Large fibroids may have local pressure effects on other organs and may interfere with pregnancy, labour or delivery. Fibroids causing trouble can be removed. In severe cases it may be best to remove the uterus (see HYSTERECTOMY).

Uterus retroversion

The UTERUS normally lies inclined forward, at a steep angle to the backward direction of the vagina. A retroverted UTERUS is one which inclines in a more backward direction so that it is directly in line with the vagina, or even bent a little backwards. Formerly most of the problems which beset women, gynaecological and otherwise, were attributed to retroversion of the uterus, but these myths have now been dispelled and the 20% or so of women whose wombs are retroverted are now considered entirely normal.

If symptoms occur in the presence of retroversion, it is possible that they are caused by a condition which is also causing retroversion. In such a case, full investigation is necessary and the cause, if any, should be corrected.

V

Vaginal bleeding (non-menstrual)

Bleeding originating in the vagina itself is uncommon, but may occur after forceful sexual intercourse. The real importance of vaginal bleeding is that bleeding, other than menstrual bleeding, may indicate cancer of the neck of the UTERUS (*cervix*), cancer of the lining of the uterus (*endometrium*) or ENDOMETRIOSIS. Vaginal bleeding after the menopause is a particularly important sign, which should never be ignored, but hormonal treatment, which combines progesterone with oestrogen, will cause vaginal bleeding. The contraceptive pill can cause occasional unexpected 'spotting' with blood and this may suggest that the dosage is incorrect.

Non-menstrual bleeding may also be due to soft polyps attached to the cervix, to inflammation of the cervix (*cervicitis*) or to the so-called CERVICAL EROSION. *Erosion* is actually due to spread of uterine lining to the outer surface of the cervix and bleeding from this cause is most likely after intercourse.

Vaginal bleeding in early pregnancy may indicate a threatened MISCARRIAGE. Later in pregnancy, bleeding may indicate separation of the placenta or the condition of placenta praevia in which the placenta lies over the outlet of the uterus.

Vaginal discharge

This is one of the commonest of women's complaints. Some degree of 'discharge' is universal and normal, the material merely being the essential mucus which is secreted by glands in the uterus and cervix and by a watery fluid that passes through the walls of the vagina from the surrounding tissues. The amount of this physiological discharge varies with the stage in the menstrual cycle and tends to be greater during pregnancy. Increased secretion is also normal in states of sexual interest or excitement.

Abnormal vaginal discharge is most commonly caused by thrush (*candidiasis*) or other yeast fungi such as monilia, much less often by infection with the *Trichomonas vaginalis* organism (*trichomoniasis*).

Vaginal trichomoniasis is fairly easily treated with Flagyl (metronidazole) and this is effective so long as the sexual partner is also treated. Vaginal THRUSH is more stubborn. The infection is encouraged by pregnancy, diabetes, antibiotics and immunosuppressive drugs or conditions and aggravated by sexual intercourse, tight clothing such as jeans, nylon underwear, poor hygiene, tampons, vaginal deodorants and other sprays, and bubble baths. Contrary to the widespread belief, the oral contraceptive pill, especially the modern low-dosage pill, does not encourage thrush.

Vaginal discharge from thrush is usually treated with long-term vaginal pessaries of an anti-fungal drug, such as miconazole, inserted daily for up to six weeks. Some experts find that pessaries used twice a week for about three months, followed by once a week usage for about nine months, is effective. Less persistent treatment seems to result in recurrence, in most cases. There has been considerable success with more recent single-dose oral anti-fungal agents and these have become popular.

Vaginal discharge is sometimes caused by a forgotten tampon which has been pushed up into the cul de sac (*fornix*) behind the cervix. Occasionally a gynaecological pessary may also be left *in situ* and forgotten.

Vaginal dryness

This is a common problem after the menopause and can lead to serious difficulties with sexual intercourse. The dryness is caused by the loss of oestrogen hormones. This loss leads to a degree of atrophy of the lining of the vagina and a reduction in its ability to transfer fluid through from the surrounding tissues. The condition can be greatly helped by the use of vaginal oestrogen creams (oestriol, marketed as Ortho-gynest or Ovestin) but persistent vaginal dryness after the menopause suggests that HORMONE REPLACEMENT THERAPY (HRT) may be a good idea.

Vaginal odour

Probably the commonest cause of this is *Gardnerella vaginalis* infection. This is a very common infection of the vagina which produces a thin vaginal discharge with a characteristic 'fishy' odour especially in the presence of a mild alkali, such as toilet soap. There are no other symptoms, but the organism, and the odour, can be sexually transmitted to the partner. The infection tends to be stubborn, but responds well to treatment with the drug Flagyl (metronidazole).

Varicose veins

Twisted, expanded and distorted veins, usually occurring in the legs, but sometimes at the lower end of the gullet (*oesopha-*

gus). Varicose veins of the legs are a misery and an embarrassment to millions, causing much distress by their unsightly appearance and the associated symptoms. Women, especially, are the victims of varicose veins and are affected more often, and more severely, than men.

Varicosity means stagnation of blood flow, poor oxygenation and nutrition to the surrounding tissues and the accumulation of metabolites which would normally be washed away and diluted by a free blood flow. The result is aching and tiredness in the legs, persistent swelling of the ankles, brownish-blue discoloration of the skin, a tendency to ulceration after minor injury and, rarely, dangerous bleeding from a ruptured vein.

The force of the heartbeat, which maintains the arterial pressure and drives the blood to all parts of the body, is almost expended by the time the blood has passed through the capillaries and reached the veins. So blood flow in the veins is passive and the pressure is very low, and this is reflected in the structure of the veins, which are thin-walled and collapse easily. Arteries have thick, elastic walls and never collapse, even when empty.

Blood returning from the head, neck and upper chest is assisted by gravity, but blood from the lower part of the body, especially the legs, has to fight gravity. A series of one-way valves in the veins allows the blood to move only in the direction of the heart, and any compression of the veins forces the column of blood to move in this direction. This external pressure is supplied by the changing shape of adjacent muscles as they contract. In the legs, most of the vein pumping is done by the calf muscles when they are contracting to extend the ankle. Interestingly, the symptoms of varicose veins are often relieved by walking.

The weight of the column of blood from the heart to the ankles is considerable and would be sufficient to cause stretching and bulging, were the veins not adequately supported by surrounding tissue. Fortunately, when all is as it should be, this heavy column of blood is broken up into sections by the valves, and its weight distributed.

The deep veins of the leg, which are large enough to carry all the returning blood, lie among the leg muscles and form an effective pump. The surface, or superficial, veins, however, lie just under the skin, are less well supported and do not receive the same all-round compressive force. These surface veins join the main deep veins up in the groin, but, at various levels in the legs, they also have cross connections to the deep veins, called the perforating veins. These, too, contain valves allowing one-way movement of blood from the superficial to the deep veins.

If the valves in the perforating veins do not close properly on back pressure, the muscle pump pressure in the deep veins is transferred to the less well-supported surface veins and the result is stretching. Once valves become leaky (*incompetent*), varicosity is inevitable. It is not known whether the primary problem is undue distensibility of the veins, so that the valves become incompetent, or whether the basis is constitutionally incompetent valves. Varicose veins tend to run in families and there is certainly a genetic tendency to one or the other of these causes – perhaps both. Other factors contribute – obesity, insufficient exercise, pregnancy, prolonged standing and local constriction from underwear elastic or garters.

Uniform, overall support, with no local tourniquet effect, can, on the other hand, be very helpful in the management of varicose veins of the legs. Well-designed and properly select-ed elastic stockings (*compression hosiery*) prevent stagnation, divert the blood into the deep veins where the muscle pump works better, prevent the reflux of blood from the deep veins and generally keep the blood flowing as it should. Stagnation is abolished, tissue nutrition improved, symptoms relieved. Even established varicose ulcers have been known to heal.

The compression should be greater at the ankle than at the thigh and should be graded along the leg. This requirement is now acknowledged by manufacturers and incorporated into the design of their products.

If compression hosiery fails, varicose veins may have to be closed off by injection of a clotting solution, or even removed altogether by the operation of stripping.

Vulva

The female external genitalia, comprising the pad of fat over the pubic bone (*mons pubis*), the two pairs of LABIA (*labia majora* and *labia minora*), the area between the labia minora, and the entrance to the vagina (*introitus*).

Vulval disorders

Because of the proximity to the anus, the vulva are always contaminated with organisms of many types. Nevertheless, inflammation (*vulvitis*) is usually controlled by natural local resistance. Vulvitis most commonly results from genital her-pes or THRUSH (*candidiasis*), especially in diabetics, but occurs also from oestrogen deficiency, or contact allergies to soaps, deodorants or traces of 'biological' washing powder remain-ing on underwear after washing. The vulva may be the site of a primary sore (*chancre*) in syphilis. Bartholinitis is inflammation of the Bartholin's glands which lie between the opening of the vagina and the labia minora. Bartholinitis may proceed to abscess formation and this may require surgical opening. Vulvovaginitis is vulvitis associated with inflammation in the vagina, and this is usually caused by candidiasis or trichomoniasis.

W

Warts (Genital)

These are essentially the same as warts anywhere else in the body and are caused by the same virus, of the papillomavirus genus of the family of papovaviruses. Genital warts are often called *condylomata acuminata*, but are just ordinary warts, all the same. They are transmitted sexually. Contact with multiple sexual partners greatly increases the chances of acquiring this unpleasant condition. Because of their location they are often more exuberant and extensive than warts elsewhere. They may spread all over the labia majora. They are usually of a cauliflower-like appearance and of a pinkish colour.

Genital warts have been of special interest because of their probable association with cancer of the cervix. Some other factor is probably also involved, however. Treatment is difficult if they are extensive, and sometimes local anti-wart applications are not sufficiently effective. Surgery under general anaesthesia may be needed.

X

X chromosome

The difference between the female and male sex is determined by the presence in every cell of the body of two X chromosomes in the female, and one X chromosome and one Y chromosome in the male. Sperm may carry either an X or a Y chromosome. If an X-carrying sperm fertilises the female egg, two X chromosomes will be present and the resulting baby will be a girl. If a Y-carrying sperm succeeds in fertilising the egg, then it will develop as a boy.

Y

Yeast
Yeasts are single-celled organisms which are classified with Fungi. In respect of women's health, the main interest arises from the strong tendency for yeast such as the *Candida* and *Monilla* species to cause THRUSH infections.

Yoghurt
Plain yoghurt has been found to be useful as a vaginal cream in the treatment of THRUSH. It restores the acidity (pH) of the vagina to a more normal level and encourages the growth of 'healthy' organisms.

Z

Z-plasty

This is a useful surgical technique extensively used by cosmetic surgeons to reduce disfiguring scars.

Zinc

Research has suggested that the metallic element zinc (Zn) may be an important nutrient for the body. Zinc deficiency is rare except in people on long-term intravenous feeding, in certain malabsorption disorders, or in ANOREXIA NERVOSA. In such cases, shortage of the element causes apathy, loss of hair, poor wound healing, eczema and diarrhoea. Recommended daily intake of zinc is 15 mg and oysters are a particularly rich source.

INDEX